KETO SWEETS AND DESSERTS RECIPES

105 LOW-CARB & FAT BOMB RECIPES FOR YOUR KETOGENIC DIET

Mary di Marzio

Contents

INTRODUCTION 5

THE HEALTH BENEFITS OF A KETO DIET 6

Cholesterol and blood pressure...6

Stable blood sugar levels 6

Losing weight...6

More energy 6

Better focus 6

Insulin resistance...7

WHAT TO EAT AND PRODUCTS ACCEPTABLE ON A KETOGENIC DIET 7

Products not allowed on a ketogenic diet:...............................7

Carbohydrate products acceptable on a ketogenic diet:.......8

HOW THE KETOGENIC DIET WORK 8

KETO RECIPES 9

INTRODUCTION

A keto diet is a low-carbohydrate diet in which the liver produces ketones that your body uses as fuel. The diet is also known as the ketogenic diet, low carbohydrate diet, or LCHF diet. The abbreviation LCHF stands for low carb high fat. The ketogenic diet is in addition to low in carbohydrates, indeed high in fat. If you eat foods that contain carbohydrates, your body produces glucose and insulin in response:

- Glucose is very easy to use as a fuel for your body. Your body prefers this when it needs energy.
- Insulin helps to absorb glucose from your blood so that your body can use it as fuel.

 The fats from your diet store your body for later use. If you eat a lot of food with much carbohydrates, your body will use it as the primary fuel source and store the fats. This boost both your weight and fat mass. If you start eating less carbohydrates, you force your body into a state of ketosis.

Ketogenic diet (ketogenic) is a high-fat diet and low carbohydrate. About 35 percent is consumed in the daily diet: fats, 50% carbohydrates, and 15% proteins. In the ketogenic diet, fat can constitute 80-90 percent of the supplied energy, and the remaining 10-20% it's a total of protein and carbohydrates.

If someone thinks that the menu of the ketogenic diet allows you to eat a large amount of fried sausages, pizza, steaks, and pork chops, yes, the ketogenic diet menu is based on fats, but on healthy and properly selected. This is a very important principle.

Carbohydrates are the body's main source of energy. When they are missing, the body begins to look for another "fuel." These are fats, specifically ketone bodies (so-called ketosis) formed in the process of fat breakdown

THE HEALTH BENEFITS OF A KETO DIET

A keto diet has many health benefits. This way, it is not only suitable for your weight, but it also gives you more energy and a better focus.

Cholesterol and blood pressure

A low-carbohydrate, high-fat diet lowers the bad LDL cholesterol, and the good HDL cholesterol rises more than a low-fat diet. Studies also show that low carbohydrate diets are beneficial for blood pressure. The keto diet is therefore suitable for your blood pressure and for your cholesterol levels.

Stable blood sugar levels

The keto diet lowers your blood sugar levels naturally by the type of food you eat. Studies shows that the diet is even more efficient than a low-calorie diet for preventing and treating diabetes.

Losing weight

Keto diet does not only helps you in weight lose because your body uses fats as its most important fuel. The level of insulin in your blood also decreases. Insulin is the hormone that provides fat storage. The keto diet change your body system into a fat-burning machine. In this way, it will help you lose weight better than low-fat and carbohydrate-rich diets.

More energy

Fats are the most efficient fuel for our bodies. That means that they provides the body with the most energy. By eating more fats, you feel more energetic throughout the day. Moreover, fats saturate better and give us a pleasantly full feeling for a long time.

Better focus

A lot of people only use the keto diet to concentrate better. Ketones are good for the brain. If you eat fewer carbohydrates, it helps to prevent spikes in your blood sugar level. This allows you to focus better and concentrate better on your work. Eating more fats also helps improves your brain function.

Insulin resistance

If insulin resistance is not treated, it can lead to type 2 diabetes. There are so many studies that show that a low-carbohydrate, ketogenic diet can reduce insulin levels to a healthy level. Other health benefits of the keto diet It is well known that the keto diet can significantly improve the health of your skin. This way, people get clearer skin, and small skin damage disappears. In addition, the keto diet has been successfully used for years for the treatment of epilepsy.

WHAT TO EAT AND PRODUCTS ACCEPTABLE ON A KETOGENIC DIET

Recipes on a ketogenic diet must be based on the right selection of ingredients. This applies to absolutely every meal. Your doctor or dietitian must decide what to eat on a ketogenic diet. However, some general principles can be considered as repetitive in this type of menu. The ketogenic diet menu should include:

- **Saturated fats,** including primarily animal fats, dairy products, and coconut oil. The ketogenic diet menu is often based on products such as pork knuckle, lard, chicken drumsticks or beef steaks;
- **Polyunsaturated fats,** obtained from fish, linseed, linseed oil, eggs, avocados, chia seeds or sesame (grains);
- **Monounsaturated fats** from nuts, olives, and olive oil.
- What to eat on a ketogenic diet is an important question, but equally important is what you do not eat when using such a diet. It is necessary to exclude some products.

Products not allowed on a ketogenic diet:

- Sweets, ice cream, jams, sweet drinks
- Grain products

- Honey
- Margarine.
- On a ketogenic diet, carbohydrates are mainly taken from vegetables and fruits.

Carbohydrate products acceptable on a ketogenic diet:
- All kinds of green vegetables with a low sugar content, including spinach and broccoli;
- Fruit (but not too much! 10 g per day is the maximum dose), e.g., apricots, raspberries, apples, plums;
- Fibber products, e.g., bran.

HOW THE KETOGENIC DIET WORK

The ketogenic diet is aimed at letting your body use fats for energy instead of carbohydrates. The carbohydrates we eat are broken down into glucose (sugar). The glucose enters the bloodstream after which it is transported to the body cells. These are, for example, the brain and muscle cells. With the ketogenic diet, you get almost no carbohydrates. This has the consequence that there is no or very little glucose in the body. Your body needs this but cannot get enough energy from the glucose for basic functions and other activities. Your body, therefore, switches to fats instead of the glucose.

KETO RECIPES

VANILLA ICE CREAM WITH HOT RASPBERRIES

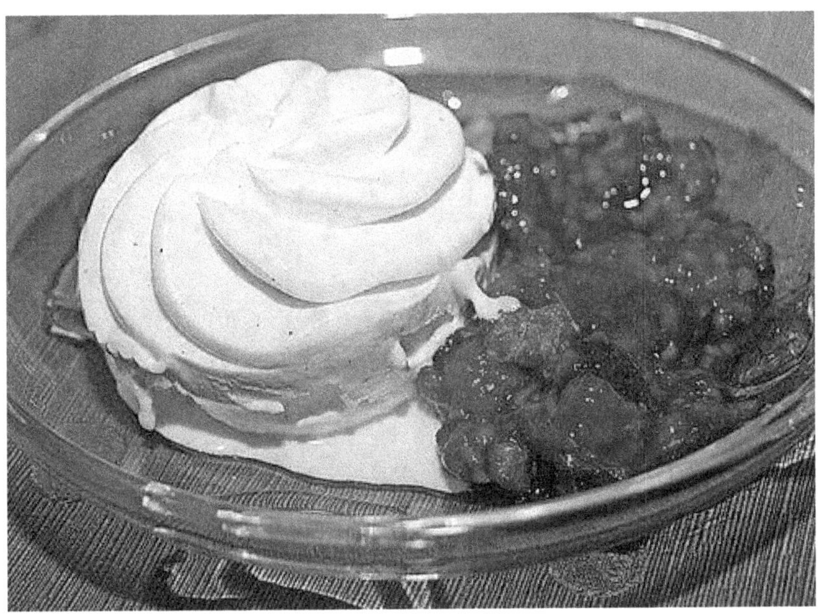

Ingredients for 1 portions

25 g   raspberries

1 ball   Ice cream (vanilla)

Preparation

Total time approx. 5 minutes

Heat the raspberries in the microwave. Put 1 scoop of ice cream on a deep plate, pour the hot raspberries over it and the delicious ice cream is ready.

RASPBERRY ICE CREAM

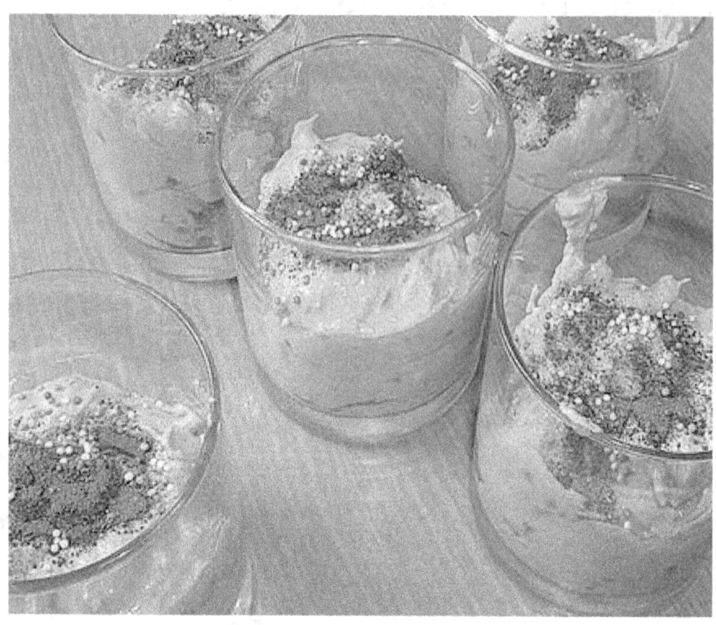

Ingredients for 1 portions

1 pck.   Raspberries,

         Powdered sugar, for dusting

500 ml whipped cream

Preparation

Total time approx. 15 minutes

Dust the raspberries in the Quick Chef with a cutting insert with icing sugar and chop them roughly. Then add the cream and continue stirring until it is a creamy mass. Transfer and place in the freezer.

LOW CARB GRANOLA MUESLI

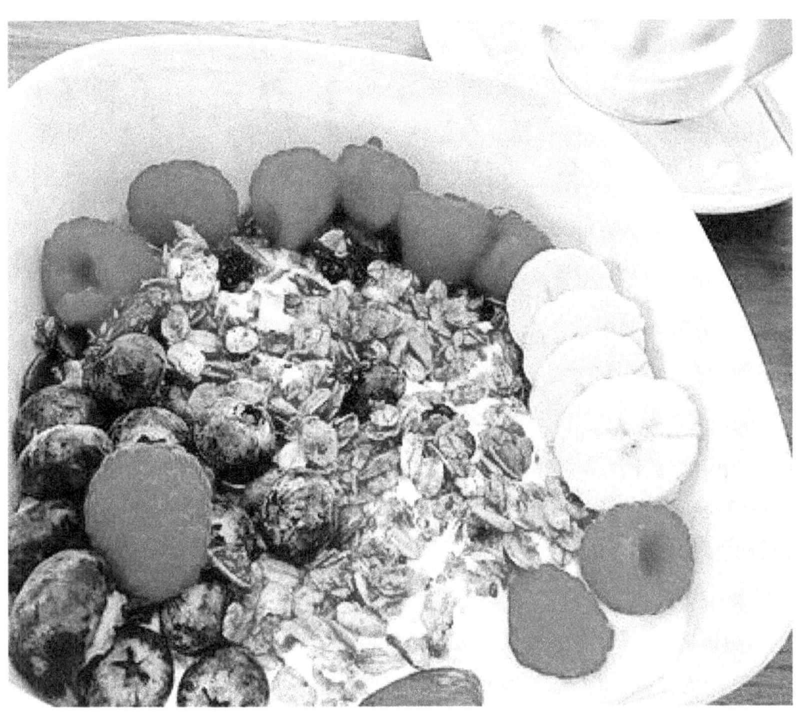

Ingredients for 1 portions

80 g	Sunflower seeds
80 g	pumpkin seeds
80 g	hazelnuts
40 g	Grated coconut or chips
80 g	walnuts
35 g	Oil (coconut, native)

60 ml   water

         Cinnamon

         Sweetener

Preparation

Total time approx. 40 minutes

Preheat the oven to 180 ° C. Chop the nuts roughly or chop them in a blender or with a blender (not too small). Heat the coconut oil in the microwave to make it liquid (this takes about 30 seconds). You can replace the coconut oil with another, heatable oil.

Then mix all ingredients. Cinnamon, alternatively cocoa, vanilla or gingerbread spice, and add liquid sweetener as desired. Attention, when tasting, the final product is a little less sweet than the "basic dough".

Place the mixture on a baking sheet lined with baking paper and press flat. Put the tin in the oven. Bake the mixture for about 30-40 minutes until it is dry and browned. In between, remove from the oven and crumble the resulting "plate" with a spoon and flatten it again. Fill the finished mass into a glass and enjoy.

The recipe results in about 10 portions of 40 g each and goes well with yoghurt or cottage cheese with fruit, but can also be eaten pure with milk. All nuts and seeds are naturally interchangeable with other varieties.

LOW CARB COCONUT ALMOND QUARK BALLS

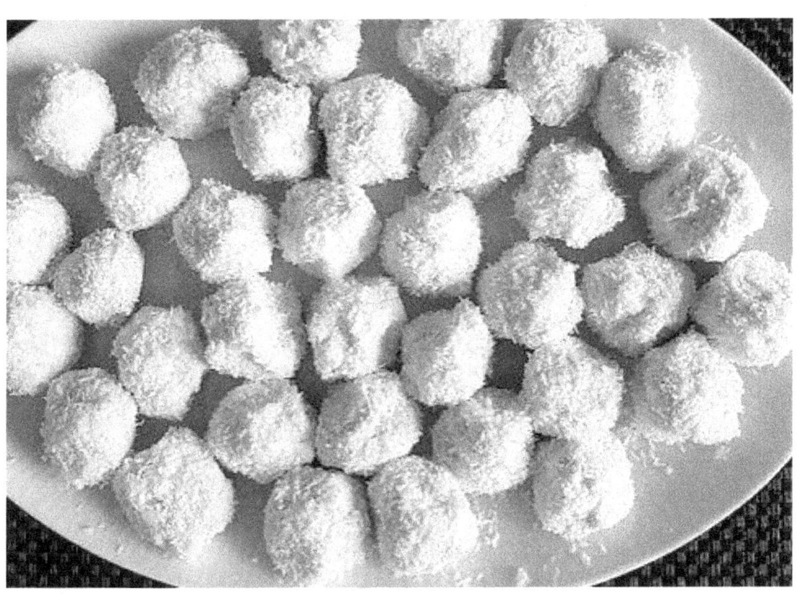

Ingredients for 1 portions

500 g   low-fat quark

100 g   Almond, peeled, about 45 pieces

50 g   Protein powder (vanilla protein powder)

100 g   Almonds, ground

60 g   Grated coconut, for the dough

100 g   desiccated coconut

Preparation

Total time approx. 4 hours 30 minutes

Mash curd cheese, egg white powder, ground almonds and 60 g grated coconut with the hand mixer to a dough mixture.

Form small balls of dough and put one almond in the middle. Roll the balls in grated coconut. If the dough balls are rather small in shape, it results in about 45 pieces. Cool the balls for at least 4 hours or overnight.

MOUSSE AU CHOCOLATE 'LIGHT'

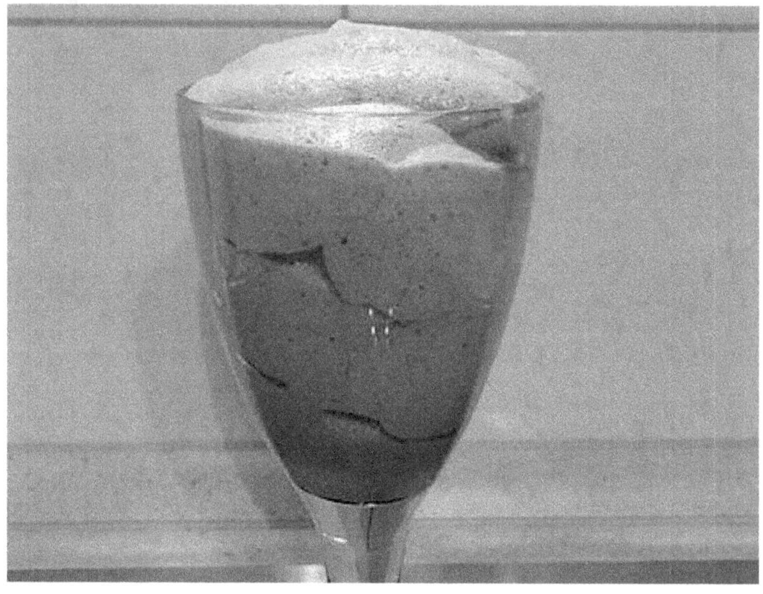

Ingredients for 1 portions

3   protein

1 tsp. heaped Cocoa powder, unsweetened

Sweetener, more fluid

Preparation

Total time approx. 3 minutes

Beat the egg whites until stiff, then add the cocoa (as desired) while stirring and add the sweetener.

Everything gives a huge portion. Although it is not comparable with real chocolate mousse, but due to the few calories a great substitute.

KILO-KILLER

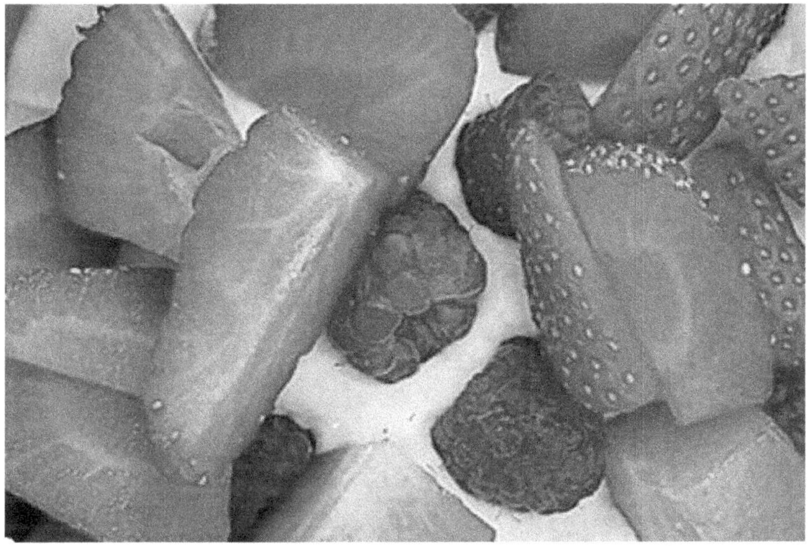

Ingredients for 1 portions

250 g   Quark

1   Egg

1 shot   Lemon juice or orange juice

          Stevia or other sweetener

1   pinch   salt

Lemon peel or orange peel, untreated, rubbed off

Preparation

Total time approx. 10 minutes

Separate the egg. Beat the egg whites with a pinch of salt to make a nice firm egg whites. Beat the egg yolks and then stir until smooth with the curds.

Add a dash of fresh lemon or orange juice, as well as the abrasion for an intense taste. Stir everything and finally fold in the egg whites. So you get a fluffy mass that saturates very well.

LOW CARB LEMON SOUFFLÉ

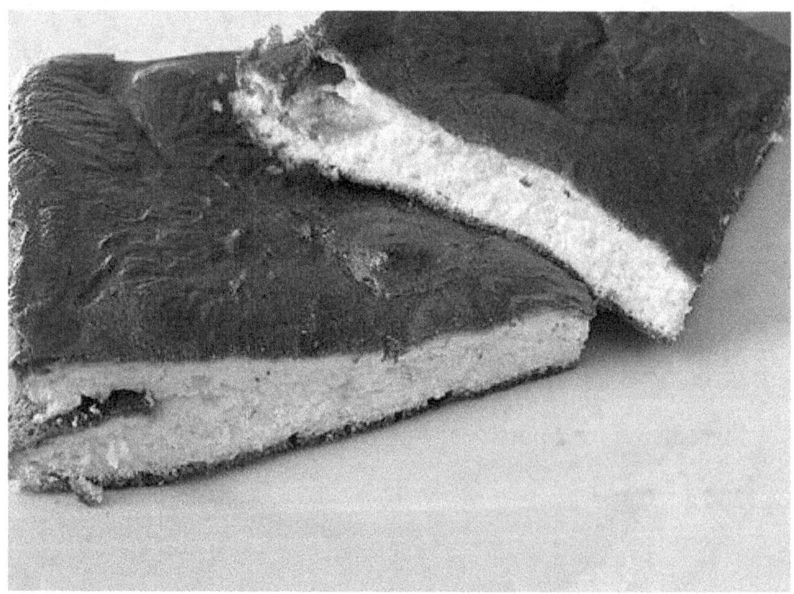

Ingredients for 4 portions

200 g   low-fat quark

2 Large Egg

4 tbsp. Protein powder, vanilla

2 tbsp. lemon juice

2 Tea spoons   Lemon peel, untreated

2 tbsp. Sweetener

Fat for the ramekins

Preparation

Total time approx. 40 minutes

Separate the eggs and beat the egg whites with a pinch of salt.

Mix the yolks with Sweetener. In the yolk mass comes now the protein powder, the quark, the lemon juice and the lemon abrasion. Stir everything into a smooth dough and then carefully fold in the egg whites, do not stir. The consistency is "fluffy".

Grease the ramekins and sprinkle with Sweetener. Spread the dough over the 4 dishes and place on a baking tray filled with warm water. The molds should be 1/3 in the water.

The soufflé is baked at 180 ° convection for 20 - 25 minutes. It should get a slightly golden yellow color.

CHOCOLATE CHIA PUDDING

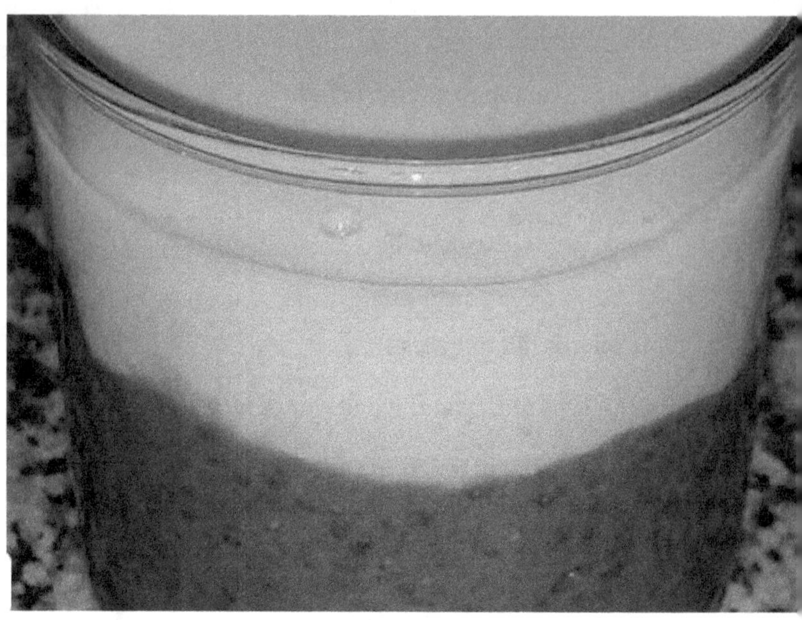

Ingredients for 2 portions

250 ml Milk or soy milk

50 ml   Soy milk (soy drink)

50 g   Chia seeds

2 tbsp. Protein powder (chocolate flavor)

2 Tea spoons   Stevia with litter (erythritol)

1 teaspoon   Back cocoa

Preparation

Total time approx. 20 minutes

Stir the milk with protein powder, cocoa and stevia. Then let the chia seeds swell in it for about 15 minutes. Then purée everything. If you do not want to wait, you can also pure it.

The pudding can also be served with custard as needed. To do this, mix vanilla protein powder with a little milk.

SIMPLE LEMON CREAM FOR CAKE

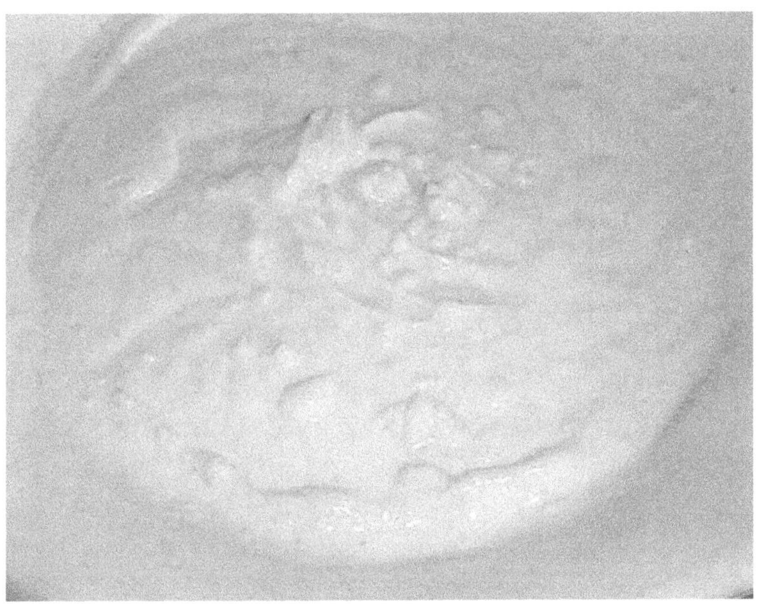

Ingredients for 1 portions

300 g   cream cheese

3 Large Lemon, untreated

1 cup   sour cream

3 tsp   Sweetener, liquid

Preparation

Total time approx. 5 minutes

Wash lemons, rub and squeeze. Put the juice, the bowl and some pulp in a bowl.

Stir in cream cheese and sour cream and sweeten with the sweetener to taste. Keep cool until use.

CHIA-CHOCOLATE PUDDING

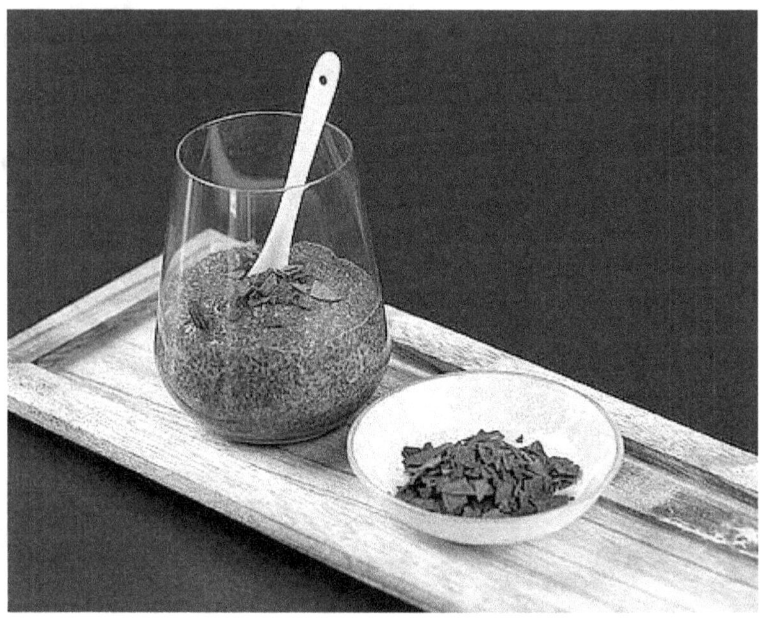

Ingredients for 1 portions

30 g   Chia seeds

180 ml coconut milk

10 g   cocoa powder

20 g   Xylitol (sugar substitute) or erythritol

Preparation

Total time approx. 1 hour 10 minutes

Mix chia seeds to make Chia Seed Flour. Then add the remaining ingredients and mix. Fill in bowls and put in the refrigerator. The stronger the consistency should be, the longer it should be cold.

CHOCOLATE CREAM LOW CARB

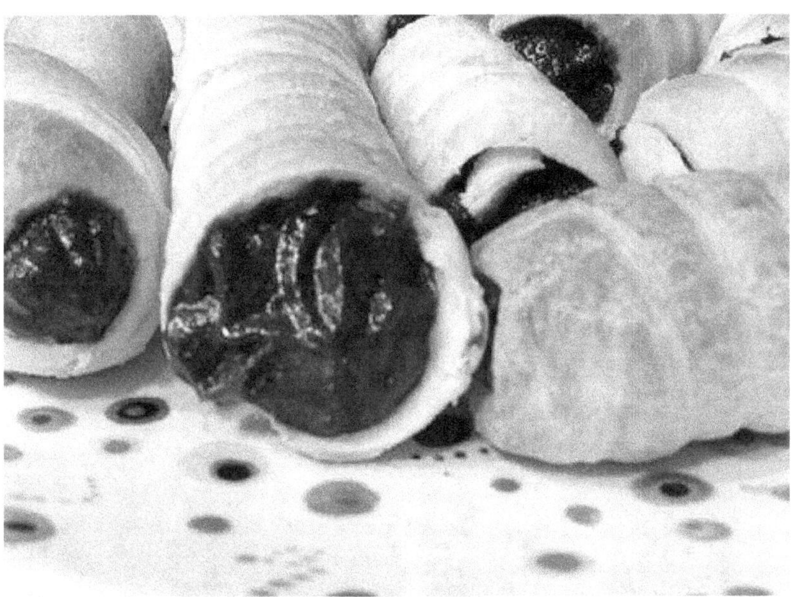

Ingredients For 1 portion

10 g   Almond, ground

5 g   Cocoa powder, unsweetened

2 g   Oil (coconut oil)

30 g   coconut milk

1 ½ tsp Sweetener (erythritol) or correspondingly less stevia

Preparation

Total time approx. 5 minutes

Mix all ingredients well. The almost 50 g make you very well fed and satisfy the lust for chocolate.

If you like it more "fluffy", you can also fold in a stiff egg whites.

ITALIAN CHEESE PLATE TO TOMATOES - CHUTNEY

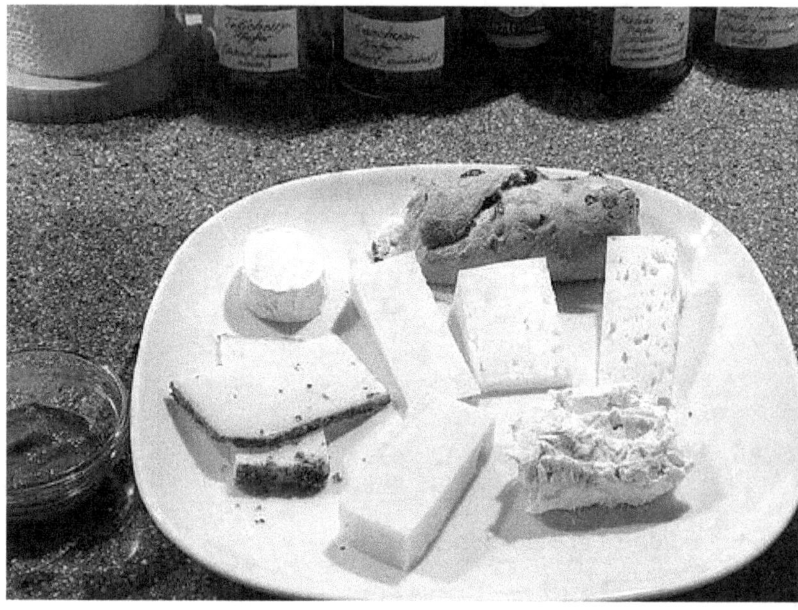

Ingredients for 8 portions

2   Tomato, (850 ml)

2   Onion

2   Garlic cloves)

30 g	Ginger, fresher
75 g	Apricot, dried200 ml	Vinegar (red wine)
	Salt
500 g	grapes
400 g	Gorgonzola
400 g	Cheese, milder
400 g	Cheese, (pecorino)
400 g	Parmesan
400 g	Cheese, (smoked provolone)
	Cayenne pepper

Preparation

Total time approx. 30 minutes

For the chutney:

Mash tomatoes and juice in a large saucepan. Peel onions, garlic and ginger, finely dice. Finely chop the apricots. All with sugar, vinegar, boil 1 tsp salt and cayenne pepper. Cook over low heat for about 3 hours. Stir more often. Taste, cool.

Wash grapes, drain. Serve cheese, grapes and chutney.

FAST PROTEIN QUARK PANCAKES

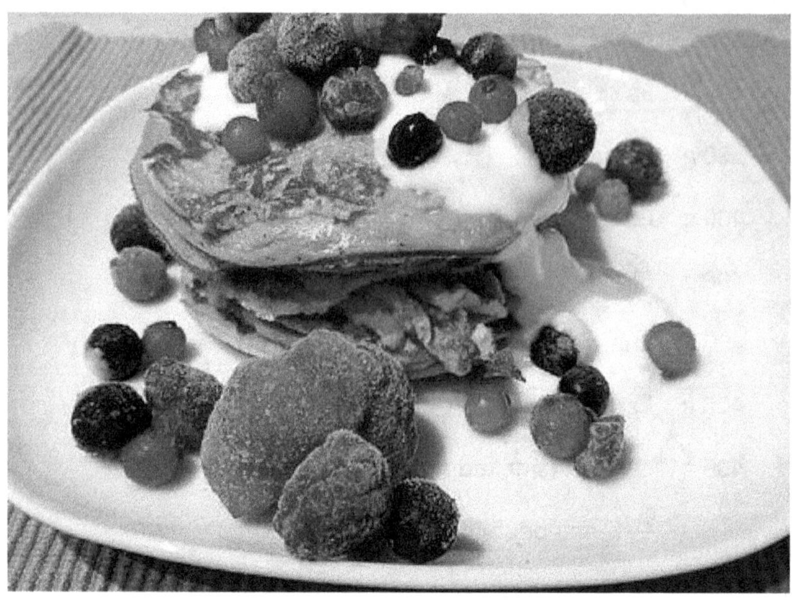

Ingredients for 1 portion

2 Large Egg

125 g   low-fat quark

30 g   protein powder

Furthermore:

    Oil

Preparation

Total time approx. 15 minutes

Mix all the ingredients in a small bowl with a whisk.

Let a pan get hot and add a small splash of oil. Bake small pancakes from the dough.

Bake the pancakes until bubbles form on the surface. Then they are ready to turn.

HOT RASPBERRIES WITH VANILLA ICE CREAM

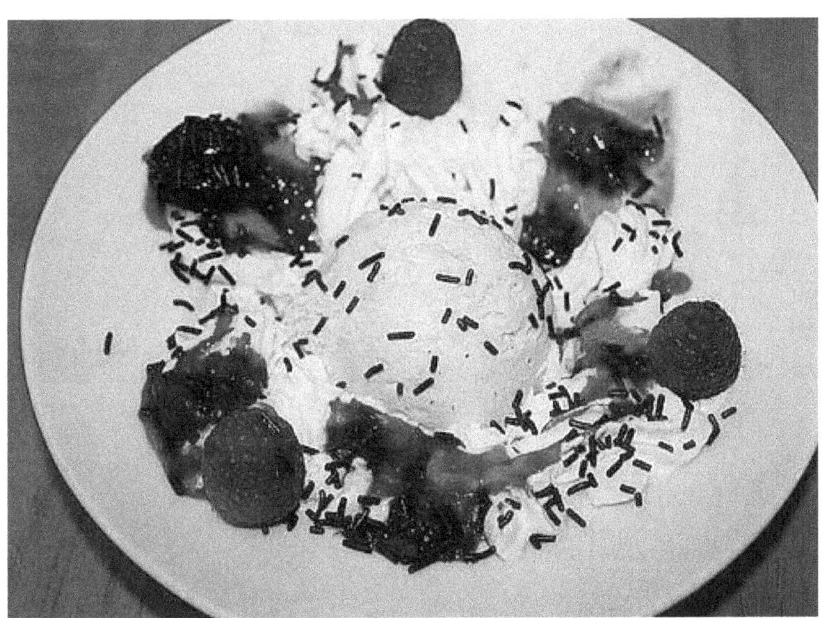

Ingredients for 1 portion

2 balls   Ice cream, vanilla

50 g   Raspberries,

Preparation

Total time approx. 4 minutes

Heat raspberries in the microwave or pan.

In the meantime, place 1-2 scoops of vanilla ice cream per serving on a dessert plate or in a glass, add hot raspberries.

RASPBERRY DREAM

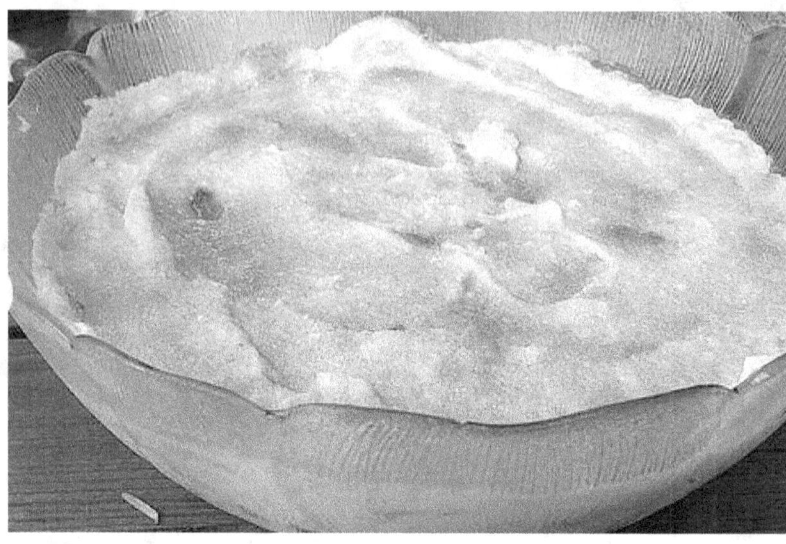

Ingredients for 4 portions

3 cups   whipped cream

2 cups   sour cream

         Powdered sugar

500 g   Raspberries, fresh or

Sugar, brown

Preparation

Total time approx. 6 hours 20 minutes

Put the raspberries in a glass bowl.

Beat the whipped cream with 2 tablespoons of powdered sugar until stiff and fold in the sour cream.

Put the cream mixture on the raspberries and finally sprinkle the brown cane sugar in a thicker layer over it.

Cover with plastic wrap and refrigerate for at least 5 hours.

AIRY-CHOCOLATEY CHOCOLATE OOPSIES

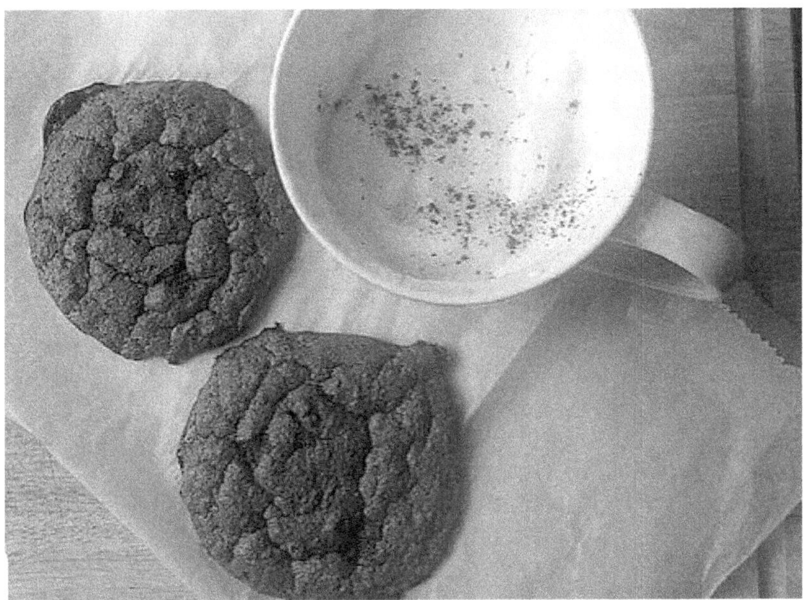

Ingredients for 4 portions

2 big   Egg

20 g   ghee

15 g   Chocolate with 99% cocoa content

       Xylitol (sugar replacement)

Preparation

Total time approx. 25 minutes

Preheat oven to 160 ° C top / bottom heat.

Separate the eggs, beat the egg whites until stiff. The egg yolk with xylitol as desired (I take up to 10 g) beat until foamy and gently under the egg white mass.

In the meantime, melt ghee with 10 g of chocolate in a small, coated pan and stir. Crush the remaining 5 g of chocolate with a grater.

Carefully lift the melted chocolate mass under the foam, then the chocolate grated.

Place four piles on a baking tray lined with baking paper. Bake in the oven for about 10 minutes until the mixture is firm, but not too brown.

MOUSSE AU CHOCOLAT LOW CARB

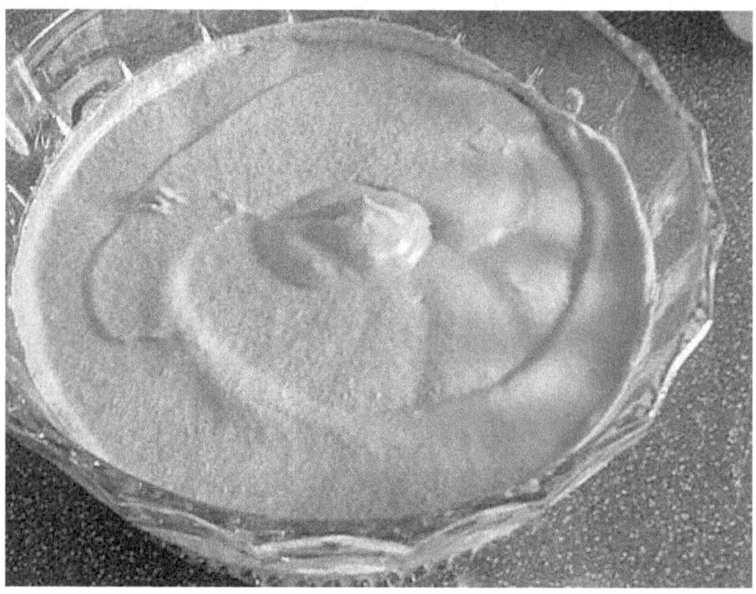

Ingredients for 4 portions

1 cup   whipped cream

2   Egg

4 tsp. heaped   Cocoa powder

            Liquid sweetener

            Aroma e.g. rum or vanilla

Preparation

Total time approx. 10 minutes

Separate the eggs.

Beat the whipped cream until stiff. Beat the egg whites until stiff. Stir the egg yolk until creamy, add cocoa powder, sweetener and flavors and stir again. Add 1 tbsp. many and cream to the chocolate mixture and stir again. Add the remaining protein and cream to the chocolate cream and fold well (do not stir) until a uniform, fluffy cream is formed.

Transfer the mousse au chocolate to a bowl or dessert bowls and, at best, refrigerate overnight in the fridge.

SMALL PANCAKES

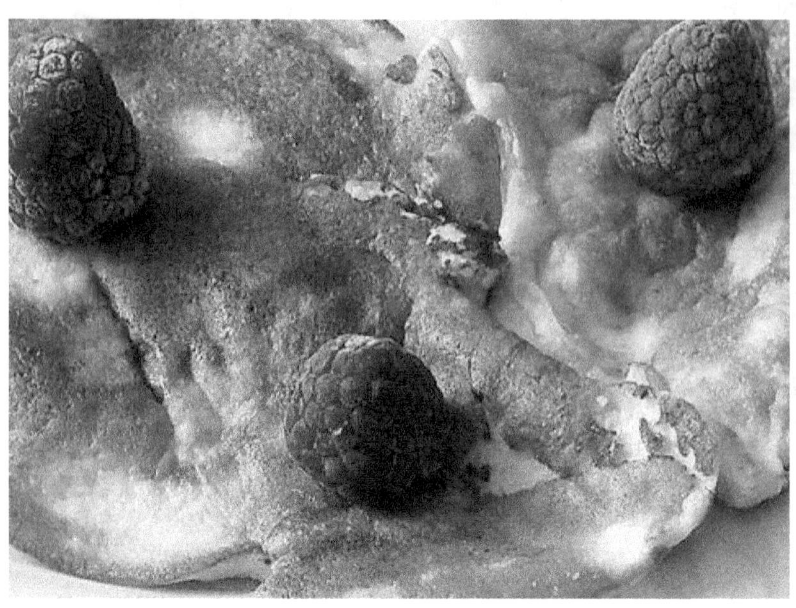

Ingredients for 1 portion

60 g   cream cheese

2   Egg

          Sweetener

Preparation

Total time approx. 7 minutes

Simply mix eggs, sweetener and cream cheese and bake small blobs in the pan with a little oil.

In my opinion the tastiest low carb pancake recipe, even if the ingredient list sounds absurd.

To save calories, I use low-fat cream cheese. The recipe can be sweetly varied with sweetener, cinnamon, baking cocoa, etc.

Also hearty taste the pancakes with some salt, pepper and herbs are delicious, here you could also take the same herb cream cheese.

APPLE BEIGNETS

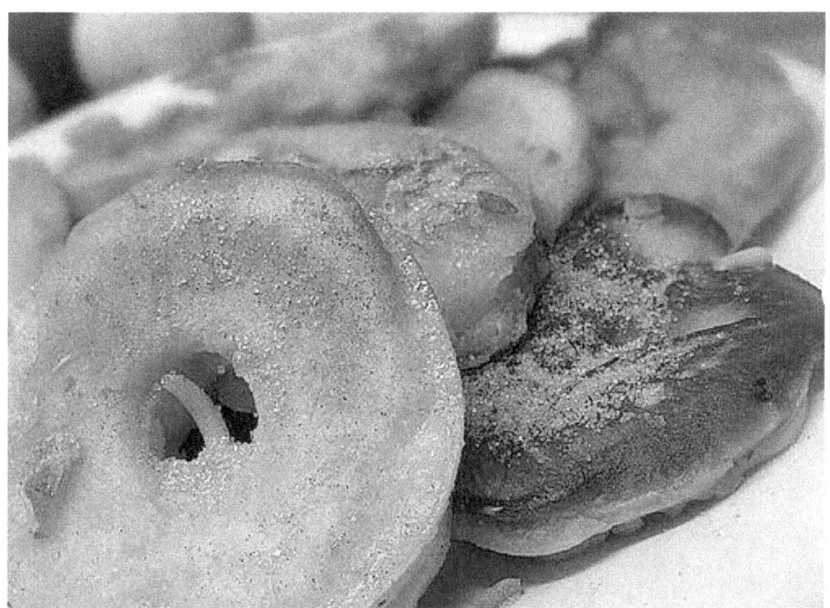

Ingredients for 4 portions

80 g   Flour

⅛ Liter cream

2   Egg

1 tsp.   salt

2   Apples

2 tbsp. Powdered sugar or

Cinnamon - sugar at will

500 g   Fat for frying

Preparation

Total time approx. 20 minutes

From the flour, the cream, the eggs and the salt stir a thick dough. Peel the apples, cut out the core and cut the apples into slices about ½ cm thick.

Heat the frying fat to 180 degrees. Pull the apple slices through the dough with a fork and turn them over. Drain briefly and bake in the hot frying fat until golden brown for 3-5 minutes. Keep the beignets warm until all the cakes have been baked.

Sprinkle with powdered sugar or cinnamon-sugar mixture before serving.

CHOCOLATE PUDDING EXTRA LIGHT

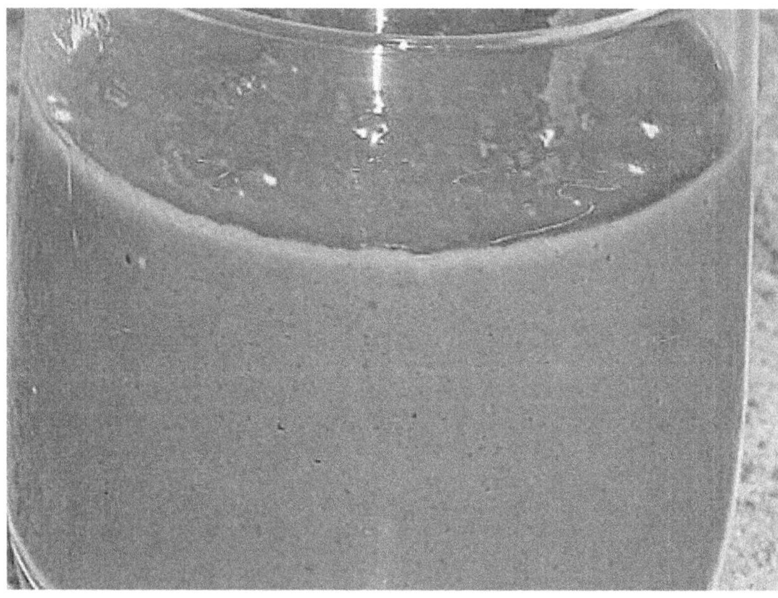

Ingredients for 3 portions

350 ml Soy milk (soy drink), light

2 Tea spoons   Cocoa powder, heavily de-oiled

        Sweetener

2 Tea spoons   Locust bean gum

        Cinnamon

        Cardamom

        Ground cloves

        Ginger, pickled

Preparation

Total time approx. 10 minutes

Put the soy milk with cocoa powder in a saucepan and stir over medium heat until the cocoa is completely dissolved. Season with sweetener. Add cinnamon, cardamom or clove powder as you like. Stir in the locust bean gum and bring to the boil while stirring.

Fill in bowls and let cool.

COFFEE FRAPPÉ

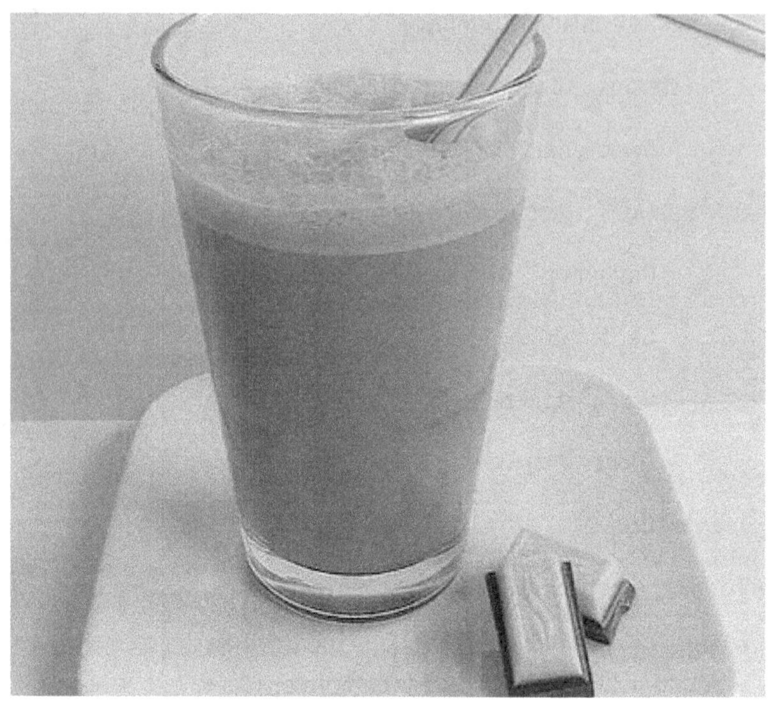

Ingredients for 1 portion

½ dl   milk

½ dl   water

2 cups   Ice cream (mocha ice cream, eg from Weight Watchers)

Preparation

Total time approx. 5 minutes

Put all ingredients in the blender and stir well.

AFFOGATO

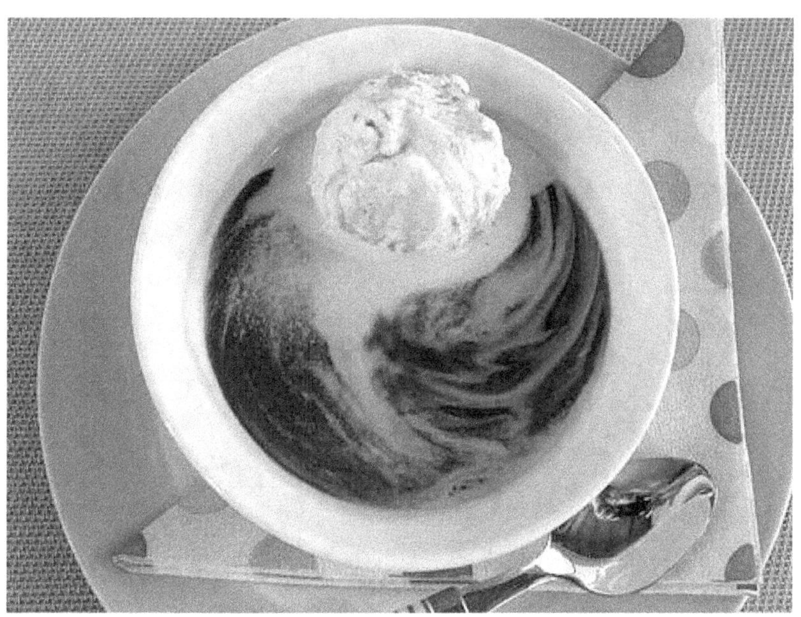

Ingredients for 1 portion

1 cup   Coffee, (hot espresso)

1 ball   Ice cream, vanilla

Preparation

Total time approx. 5 minutes

Put a scoop of vanilla ice cream in a coffee cup and pour the hot espresso over it.

This small "iced coffee" is ideal as a dessert or as a small Italian refreshment.

RASPBERRY AND MASCARPONE DESSERT

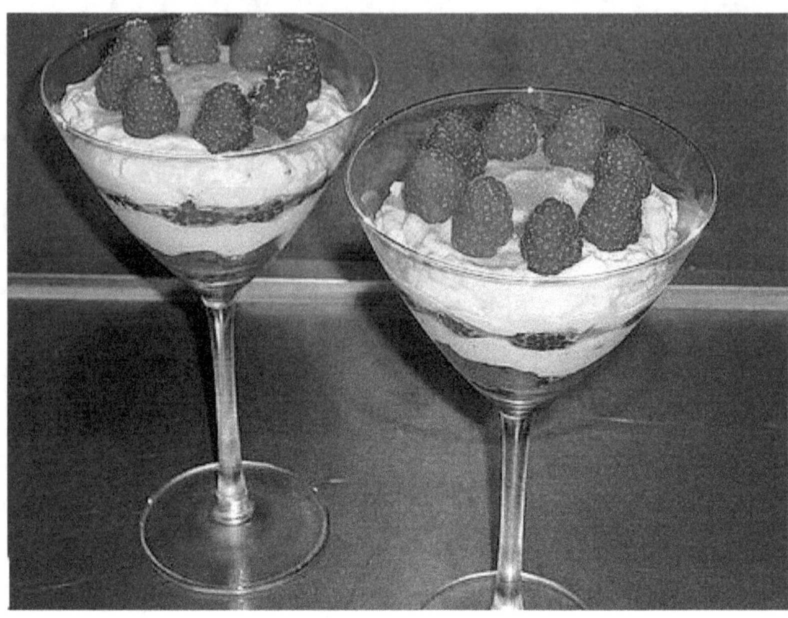

Ingredients for 6 portions

600 g   Raspberries, fresh or frozen

500 g   mascarpone

100 ml coconut milk

50 g   desiccated coconut

1   Vanilla pod vanilla sugar

Sugar, brown

Preparation

Total time approx. 10 minutes

If necessary, the raspberries are thawed in the sieve and placed in a casserole dish or the like at the bottom Spread. Glass is especially pretty here because you can see the layers.

The mascarpone is stirred smoothly with the coconut milk, the coconut flakes, the vanilla pulp and vanilla sugar and then poured over the raspberries. Finally, brown sugar is sprinkled over the cream, creating a sweet layer.

OAT DESSERT

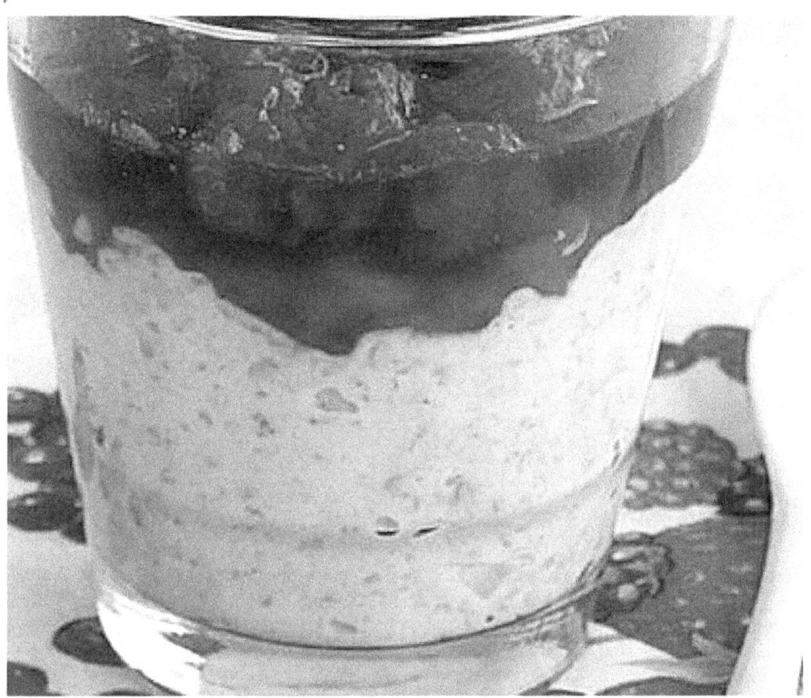

Ingredients for 1 portions

50 g   Oatmeal, meaty

250 ml Milk (0.1% fat)

1 tbsp.   Cream cheese (<20% fat)

2 tbsp.   low-fat quark

          Sweetener, liquid

          Vanilla flavor or vanilla

Preparation

Total time approx. 15 minutes

Boil the milk with the oatmeal on medium heat, stir and cook a porridge. When the porridge is ready, turn off the oven and fold in the cream cheese. Finally add the lean quark. Season with vanilla flavor and sweetener.

VANILLA ALMOND PUDDING

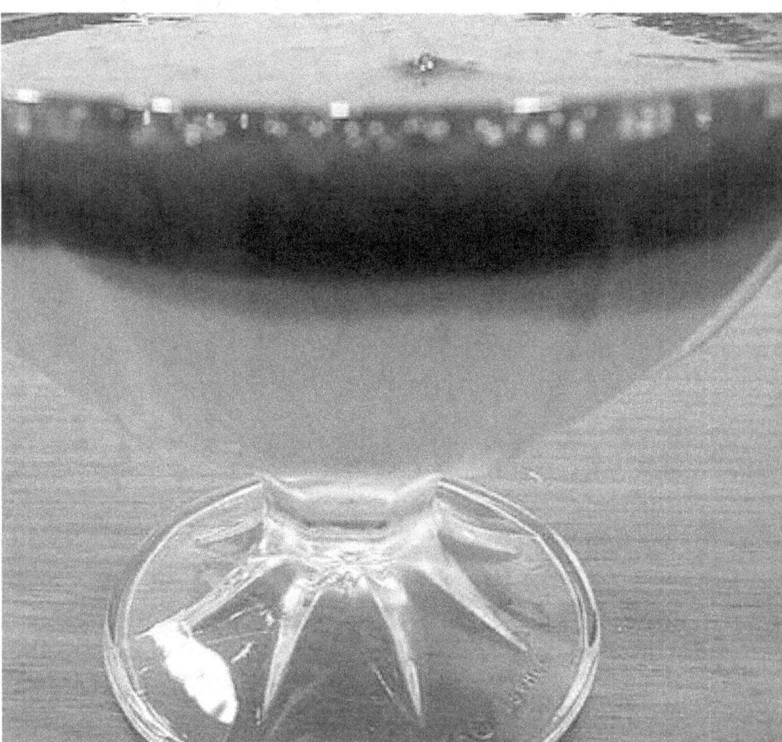

Ingredients for 4 portions

200 ml Almond milk (almond drink), unsweetened

300 ml cream

1   Vanilla pod, fresh

1 pck.   Gelatin, ground

1 tbsp. Water, cold

4 g   Sweetener.

           Liquid sweetener as needed

1   Yolk, if required

Preparation

Total time approx. 55 minutes

Slit the vanilla pod lengthways, press it apart and scrape off the vanilla pulp with the back of the knife. Mix the vanilla pulp and the liquid cream well.

Stir the gelatin in a microwave-proof bowl with 1 tbsp. Cold water and let it swell for a few minutes. In the meantime, warm the almond milk in the microwave for 1 min.

Also heat the gelatin in the microwave for about 1 min until it melts. Slowly pour the warmed almond milk into the gelatin, stirring continuously. Stir everything well, there must be no more gelatin lumps. If this is the case, heat the mass briefly in the microwave again and stir well again.

Add the cream with the vanilla pulp and sweeten with the sweetener. Sweeten to taste with some liquid sweetness. Now carefully stir in the egg yolk, which gives the pudding a nice vanilla-yellow color.

Fill the vanilla almond cream in 4 small serving dishes and refrigerate. After 15 - 20 minutes you can gently stir the mass, so that prevents the vanilla mark settles on the ground. Then let it solidify in the fridge for at least 30 minutes.

LOW CARB PUDDING

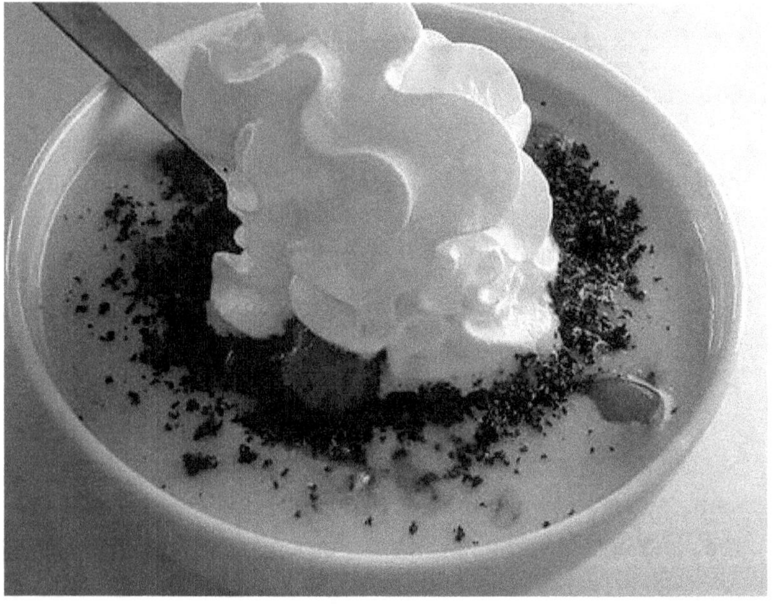

Ingredients for 4 portions

500 ml Soy milk (soy drink), unsweetened

1 teaspoon, heaped   guar Gum

1 tbsp. Cocoa powder, de-oiled

1 kl. Bottle   Vanilla flavor or 1 vanilla pod

        Sweetener

Preparation

Total time approx. 25 minutes

Put the soymilk into a saucepan, sift the Guar Gum very slowly and stir quickly with a whisk, otherwise the lump will give. Let it swell for 10 - 15 minutes.

Then you add sweetener (liquid) as needed, as well as the vanilla flavor. It is conceivable as back flavor or like real vanilla (a pod). If you do not mind the 8 g extra KH, you can also add a bag of vanilla sugar. Then go to 1-2 - stir in the cocoa powder thoroughly.

Then slowly heat and stir constantly. The cocoa powder dissolves well and the guar gum binds better.

Serve the pudding warm or cold. When it is allowed to cool, stir occasionally. For extra creaminess, you can also treat the pudding with a blender to mix everything.

APPLE QUARK CINNAMON DESSERT

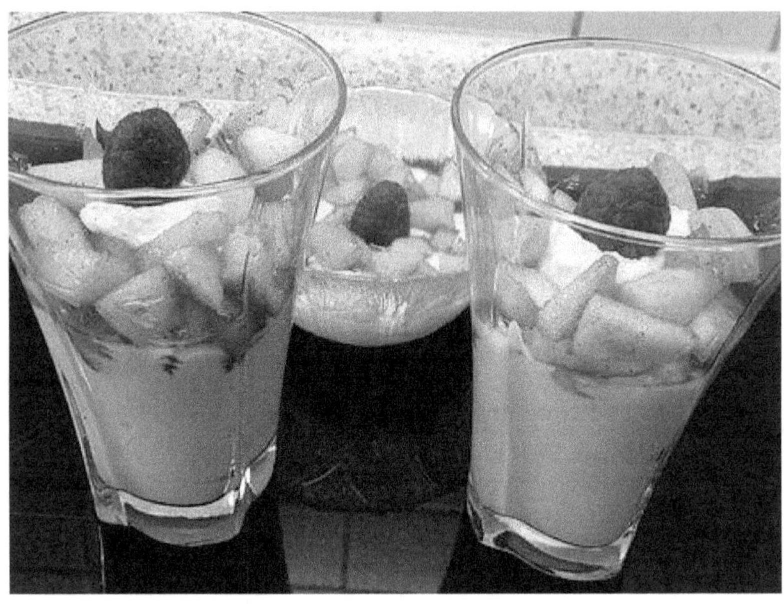

Ingredients for 2 portions

250 g   Quark 20% or skimmed quark

2   apples

1 teaspoon   butter

2 tbsp. Xylitol (sugar substitute) or sugar

           Cinnamon

           Cream cheese

Preparation

Total time approx. 20 minutes

Peel and core the apples first. These then cut into about 1 cm pieces.

Then melt the butter in a pan (I take salted, this brings out the taste better). If it has become liquid, add the sugar. Start to brown the liquid, add the small apple and caramelize everything together.

Meanwhile, mix the quark with a little sugar and fill in small jars or bowls.

When the apple pieces turn slightly brown, add a pinch of cinnamon (can be more). Continue to brown for another 1 - 2 minutes.

Distribute the pieces of apple on the quark and finally a dollop of cream cheese as a topping on top.

BAVARIAN CREAM LOW CARB

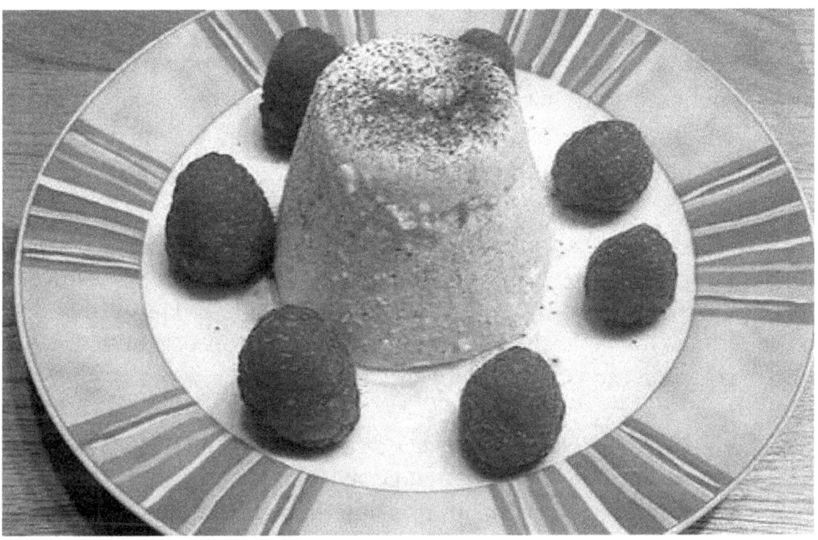

Ingredients for 6 portions

400 ml milk

6 leaves   Gelatin, white

Water, cold for soaking

4   Egg yolk, from very Fresh eggs

1   Vanilla pod

200 ml cream

20 drops   Stevia, liquid

          Ice cubes

Preparation

Total time approx. 4 hours 30 minutes

Soak the gelatin leaves in a bowl of cold water for at least 10 minutes. Slit the vanilla pod lengthwise and scrape the pith out with the back of the knife. Let the scratched peas together with the vanilla cheese and the milk in a saucepan get hot.

For the hot water bath put a metal bowl (preferably with a round bottom) in a pot with water. The bowl must hang in the pot so that its bottom touches the water, but not the bottom of the pot. Put both together on the stove so that the water can boil.

Add the yolks and the liquid stevia to the bowl and stir until frothy. Remove the vanilla pod from the milk and pour the vanilla milk into the egg yolk. Always stir vigorously until the cream in the water bath becomes warm and viscous.

For the cold water bath in a large bowl, mix cold water with some ice cubes. Put the metal bowl with the egg yolk cream in it. Drain the gelatin leaves one at a time and stir individually under the warm cream until they dissolve.

Then stir the cream for some time. Now beat the cream until stiff and use a whisk to carefully lift it under the cream as soon as it starts to gel.

Briefly rinse out six little molds (approx. 200 ml each) with cold water and drain before filling in the cream. Then put the dishes in the refrigerator for at least 4 hours.

LOW CARB QUARK BAGS

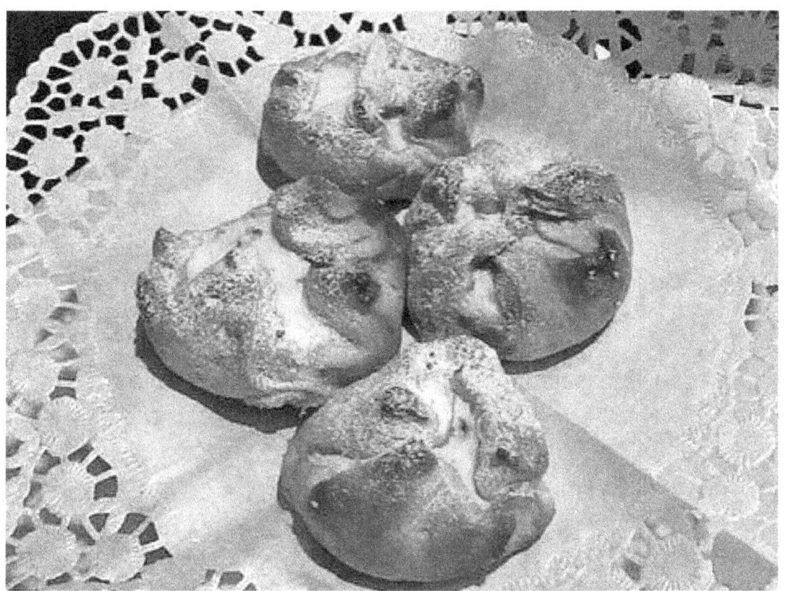

Ingredients for 1 portion

150 g   soy flour

150 g   chickpea flour

300 g   Wheat flour, Type 405

4   Egg

1 cube yeast

1 teaspoon   honey

3 tablespoons, heaped Stevia

500 g   Lean quark, 0.3% fat

1 tbsp. raisins

50 ml   Oil, tasteless, z. As rapeseed oil or sunflower oil

100 ml milk

1 tsp.   salt

Preparation

Total time approx. 1 hour 50 minutes

Crumble the yeast in a large bowl. Mix with 100 ml of lukewarm milk and approx. 150-200 ml lukewarm water. Add the honey and stir gently. Leave to rise in a warm place until the yeast has formed small flowers on the surface of the liquid.

Mix the wheat flour with soy and chickpea flour, 1 pinch of salt and 1 tablespoon of stevia and add to the yeast mixture. Add 1 egg and the egg white from the second egg to the flour and knead into a smooth, elastic dough.

Put the egg yolk in a bowl and, if desired, mix with 1/2 teaspoon vanilla sugar. This is needed at the end for brushing. If the dough is too sticky or liquid add some soy or wheat flour.

Distribute the oil on the work surface and knead the dough again with your hands. You can also take a little less oil. Form the dough into a ball, cover with a clean cloth and leave to rise in a warm place until the volume has doubled.

For the quark filling, mix the quark with 2 tablespoons stevia, 2 eggs and raisins.

Knead the dough again, split into 2 halves, roll out approx. 1 cm thick each and cut into 12 squares with a pizza cutter. Put about 1 teaspoon of the curd cheese cream on each square, fold the corners to the middle and press lightly so that small packages are formed. Place the packets with sufficient distance from each other on a baking sheet covered with baking paper. Brush with egg yolk and bake in the oven at 180 ° C in 15 - 20 minutes until golden brown.

Then allow to cool and, depending on your taste, dust with stevia or powdered sugar.

LOW CARB PROTEIN QUARK DESSERT

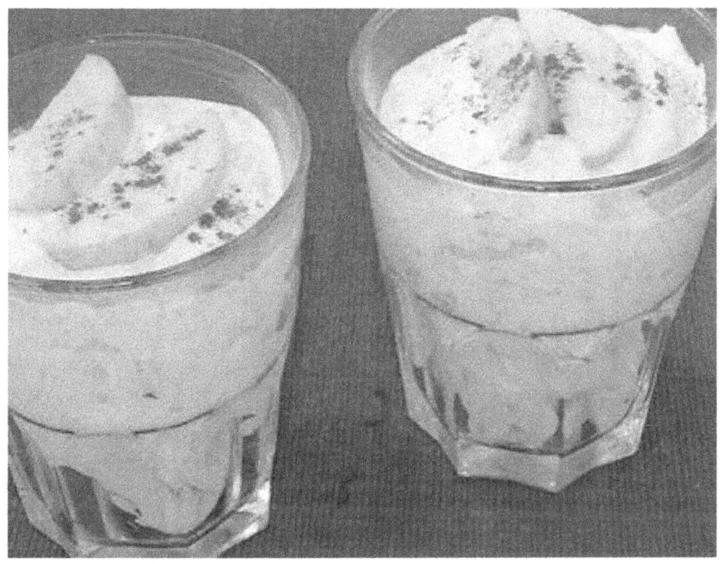

Ingredients for 4 portions

350 g   Yogurt

500 g   low-fat quark

30 g   Protein powder, , for example, vanilla

        Fruit. E.g. apples

        Flavdrops

Cinnamon

Preparation

Total time approx. 10 minutes

Put all ingredients in a bowl. Mix everything well, so that the protein powder is dissolved. Mix with flavdrops, cinnamon or fruit as desired.

LOW CARB CHIA SCHOCOFFEE PUDDING

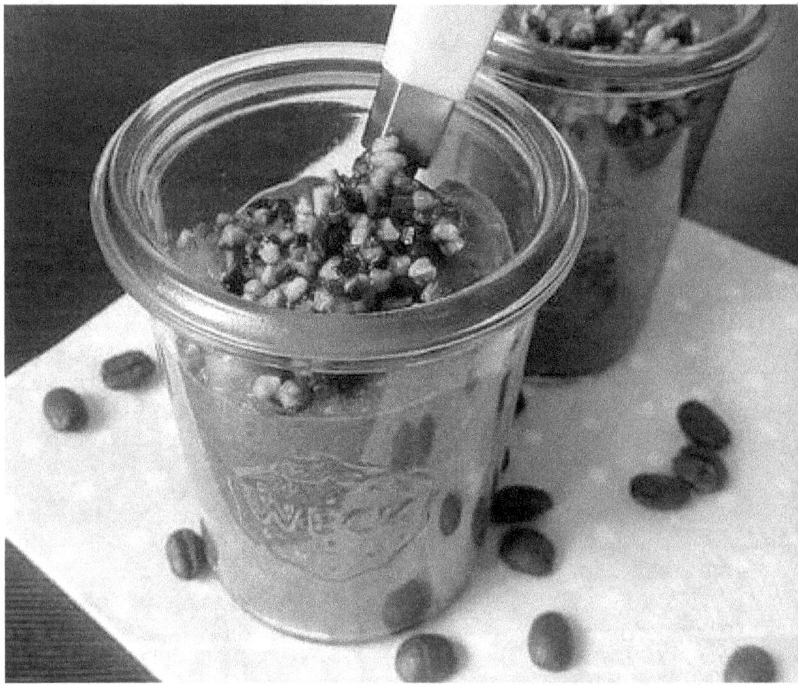

Ingredients for 1 portion

30 g   Chia seeds

60 ml   coconut milk

120 ml Coffee, cold

10 g   cocoa powder

20 g   Xylitol (sugar substitute) or erythritol

Preparation

Total time approx. 10 minutes

Mix the chia seeds to make chia seed flour. Add the remaining ingredients and mix further.

The firmer you like the texture, the longer it will stay cold.

Enjoy!

LOW CARB RASPBERRY DESSERT

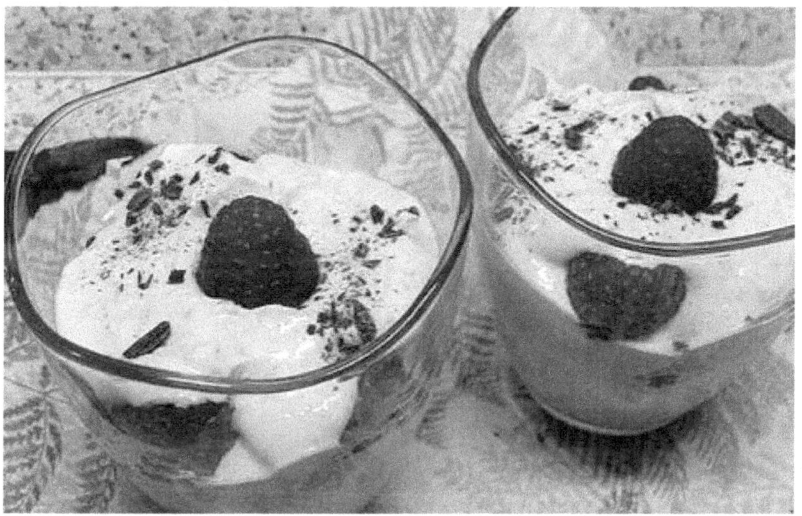

Ingredients for 2 portions

100 g   Cream cheese, natural

200 g   Quark (20%)

20 g   Xylitol (sugar substitute), possibly more

80 g   raspberries

1 ½ tbsp.   Chocolate, dark (75%), grated

¼ tsp.   vanilla powder

Preparation

Total time approx. 5 minutes

Mix cream cheese, quark and xylitol well until the xylitol dissolves. Approximately Stir in 2/3 of the raspberries or even lightly crush them, the quark will taste more aromatic. The coarsely grated chocolate, it may be quiet coarse pieces, and stir in the vanilla.

Fill in 2 small dessert glasses and decorate with the remaining raspberries and a few chocolate rasps.

BLACKBERRY COCONUT DESSERT

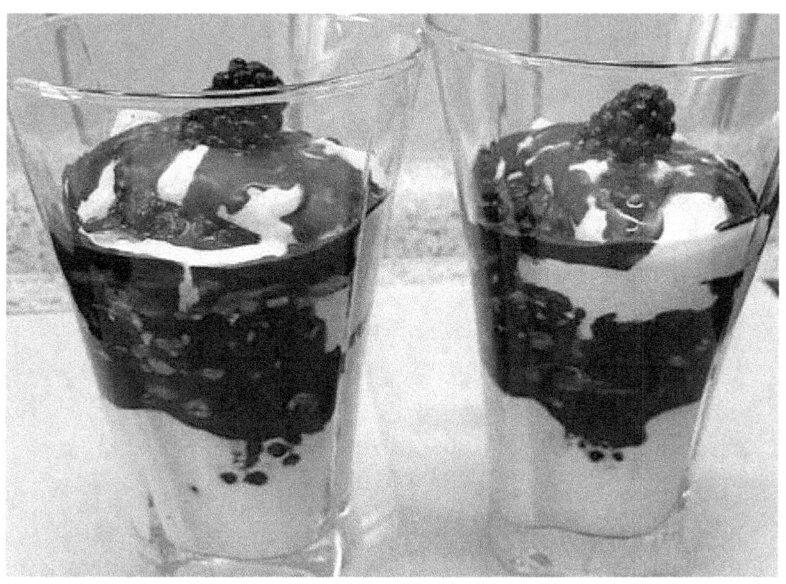

Ingredients for 2 portions

340 g   Yoghurt, Greek (10%, cow's milk)

1 ½ tbsp.   Erythritol (sugar replacement), alternatively
xylitol, to taste more

2 ½ tbsp.   coconut flakes

1 small bowl   Blackberries, other berries

¼ tsp   Vanilla, ground

In addition: for the production of chocolate:

25 g   coconut oil

20 g   cocoa

1 tsp.   Erythritol (sugar replacement)

Preparation

Total time approx. 2 hours 11 minutes

Mix yoghurt, erythritol, vanilla and coconut flakes well, so that the sugar dissolves. Wash berries and drain well.

In a small pot, melt the coconut oil, dissolve erythritol in it and stir in the cocoa with a whisk. Remove from heat.

Prepare dessert glasses and add some yogurt mixture, add some blackberries. The chocolate mixture spoon wise, about 2 tablespoons, give it. Then refill yoghurt, blackberries and chocolate layer by layer. Finally, add some chocolate and decorate it with a berry. Put in the refrigerator for about 2 hours. The chocolate then hardens.

Approximately remove from the refrigerator 10 - 15 minutes before serving.

It can be kept for at least 3 days.

LOW CARB DESSERT WITH FRESH MANGO

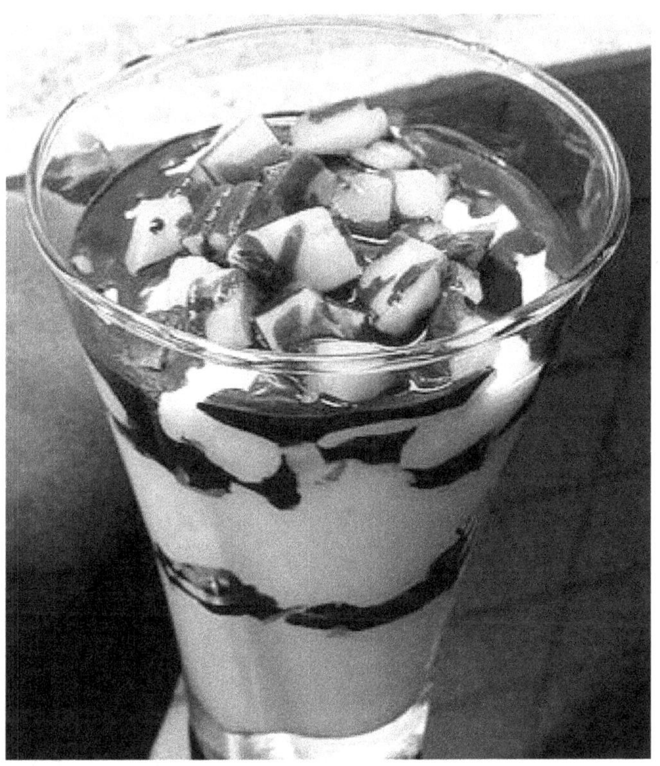

Ingredients for 4 portions

1   Mango, fresh, ripe

680 g   Yogurt, Greek (10%), made from cow's milk

5 tbsp. coconut flakes

4 tbsp. Erythritol (sugar substitute), alternatively xylitol

½ tsp.   vanilla

In addition: for the production of chocolate:

40 g   coconut oil

35 g   back cocoa

1 tbsp. Erythritol (sugar substitute), alternatively xylitol

Preparation

Total time approx. 2 hours 11 minutes

Mix the yoghurt, erythritol, vanilla and coconut flakes well so that the sugar dissolves. Peel the mango and cut the top in cubic shape (first longitudinal, then cross sections). Cut right across the core with a knife from right to left. This is how the cubes fall off. Do the same with the underside.

In a small pot melt the coconut oil, dissolve erythritol in it and stir in the cocoa with a whisk. Remove from heat.

Prepare dessert glasses and add a little yoghurt mixture, put a few mango cubes on top. The chocolate mixture spoon wise, about 2 tablespoons, give it. Then yogurt, mango and chocolate in layers again. Finally, a layer of yogurt and mango cubes. Decorate with the remaining chocolate. Put in the refrigerator for about 2 hours. The chocolate then hardens.

Approximately remove from the refrigerator 10 minutes before serving.

BLACKBERRY AND APPLE DESSERT

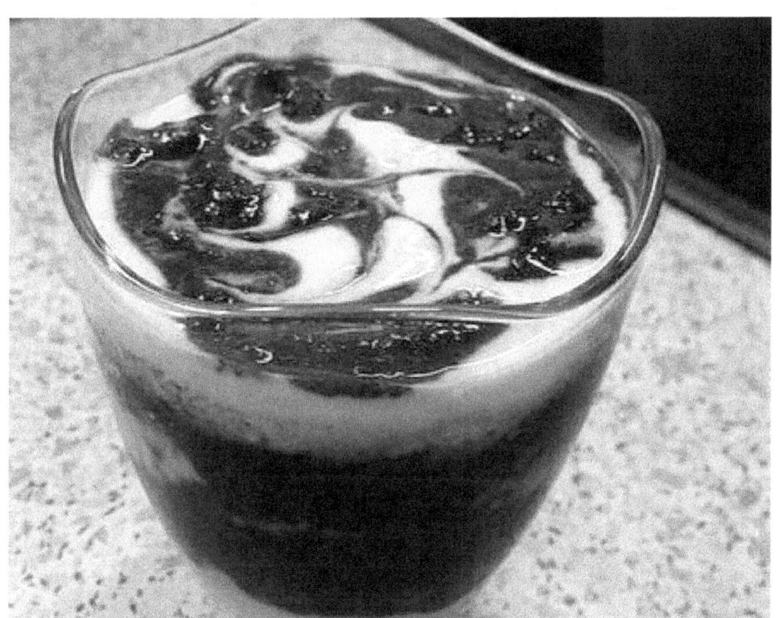

Ingredients for 2 portions

130 g blackberries

50 g Apple without core casing

6 tsp Erythritol (sugar substitute), bronze

350 g Natural yoghurt

¼ tsp. cinnamon

Preparation

Total time approx. 10 minutes

From the apple 50 g, like with shell, finely grate or grate. If necessary, rinse off the blackberries for a short time. Mash both in a jar of erythritol bronze and cinnamon. Taste, if still sweetness is missing.

Layer in jars alternately, natural yoghurt, blackberry-apple, etc., make about 3 layers. The top layer should be blackberry-apple. Decorate with the help of a wooden stick.

LEAN PUDDING CREAM LOW CARB

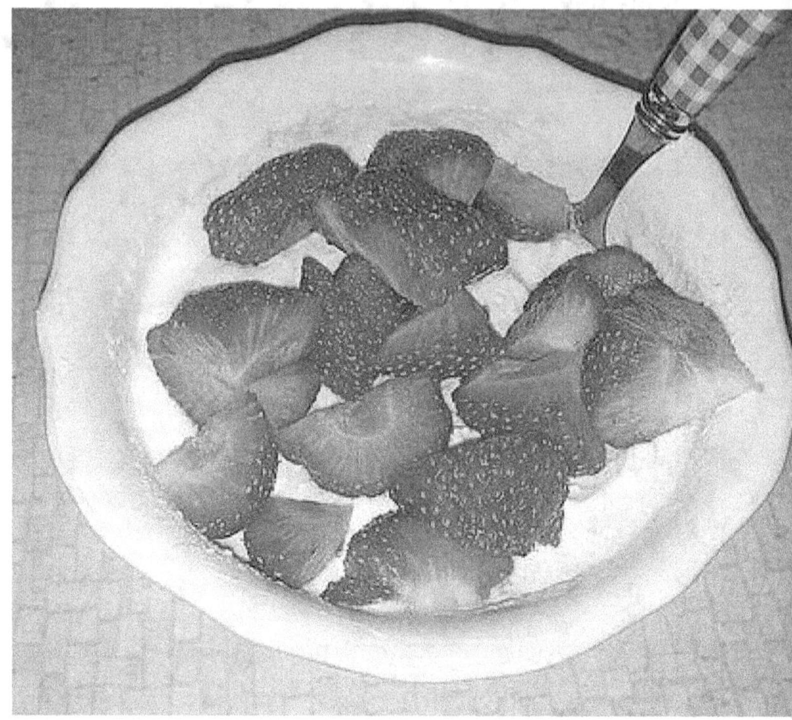

Ingredients for 1 portion

250 g   low-fat quark

            Berries, z. B. strawberries, blueberries

            Sweetener

150 ml water

1 tbsp. Oil, (linseed oil), optional

30 g   Nuts, (Brazil nuts), optional

50 g   Oatmeal, optional

Preparation

Total time approx. 10 minutes

Wash berries. Put the curds, water and berries in a blender, sweeten with sweetener and mix. Optionally, an oil of linseed oil can be added or 30g Brazil nuts. If the cottage cheese cream is eaten for breakfast, you can add oatmeal. This is a good cereal substitute.

FITNESS DESSERT APPLE CINNAMON SKINNY QUARK

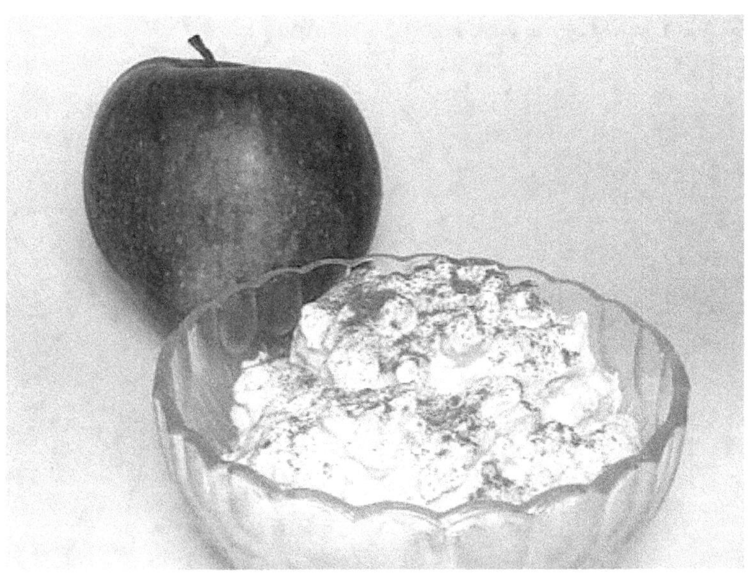

Ingredients for 2 portions

1 tbsp. Mesquite powder (sweetener)

1 tbsp. cocoa powder

250 g	low-fat quark
1	Apple
	Stevia powder
	Cinnamon
Little	lemon juice

Preparation

Total time approx. 5 minutes

Peel the apple, core it and cut it very finely.

Put cocoa, mesquite powder and cottage cheese in a bowl and mix to a homogenous mass. Add the apple pieces and stir again. Season with stevia, cinnamon and lemon juice.

LOW CARB CHOCOLATE PUDDING WITHOUT PROTEIN POWDER

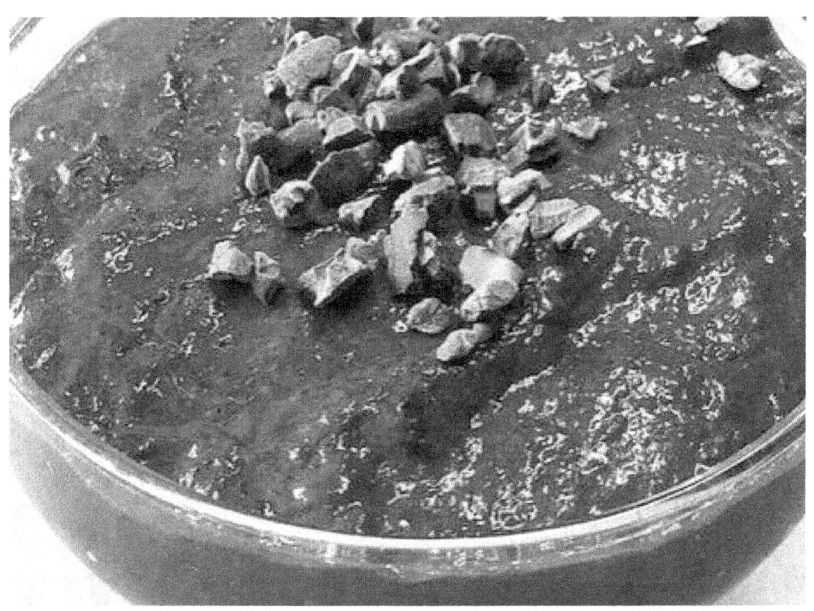

Ingredients for 1 portion

3 tsp   back cocoa

3 tsp   Xylitol (sugar substitute) light

250 ml Plant milk (vegetable drink)

1 tbsp. butter

Possibly.   Liquid sweetener

Preparation

Total time approx. 7 minutes

Mix the baking cocoa and the Xucker light and mix with the cashew milk. Then heat everything in the pot. Bring to a boil. Remove from the plate, stir in the butter and let melt.

Depending on the desired consistency, stir in 2 or 3 lightly heaped TL psyllium husks and let them swell for one minute. Season with liquid sweetener.

The cashew milk can of course be replaced by any other milk, but cashew milk tastes good and has very little carbohydrate.

LOW CARB MELON DESSERT

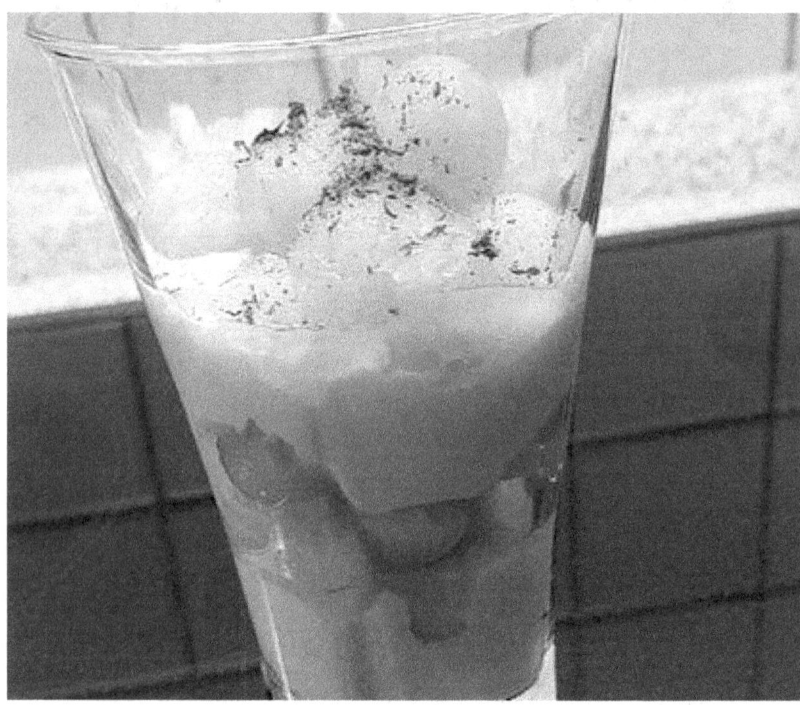

Ingredients for 2 portions

250 g   Quark, 40%

150 g   Yogurt, 3.8%, creamy

½   Gallia melon

1 ½ tbsp. Sugar substitute (raw cane sugar substitute), substitute erythritol

Ground cinnamon

Preparation

Total time approx. 5 minutes

Quark, yogurt, sweetener and cinnamon and season to taste.

Core the Gali-melon and cut out in a spherical shape or cut into small pieces. Layer in a glass.

This dessert should no longer be left standing, as the melon could possibly water down the quark.

Those who do not need low carb can also use brown sugar as a sweetener. Possibly. Decorate with grated, dark chocolate.

LOW CARB CHOCOLATE DESSERT

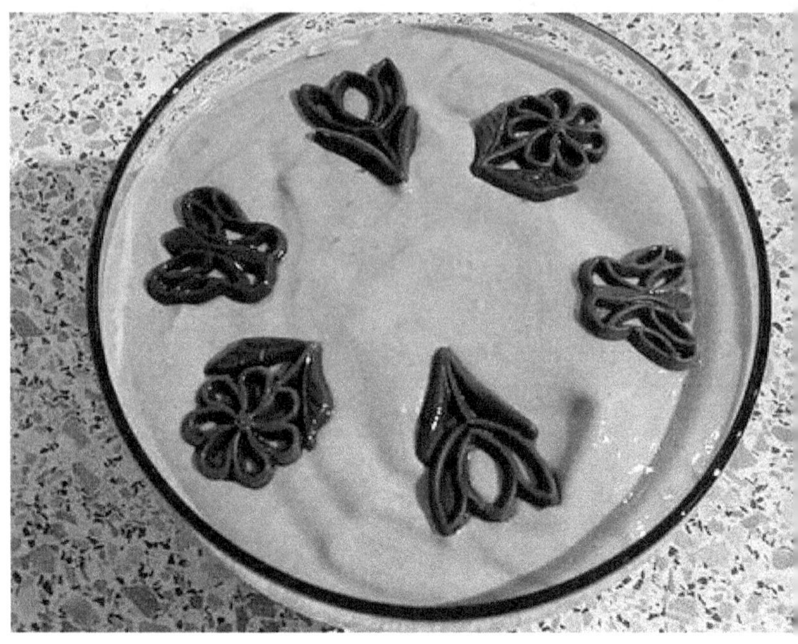

Ingredients for 1 portion

250 g   Quark with 20% or 40% fat content

2 tbsp. Back cocoa

2 splashes   Sweetener or vanilla flavedrops

Preparation

Total time approx. 5 minutes

Mix all ingredients together. Season with sweetener.

LOW CARB PANCAKES

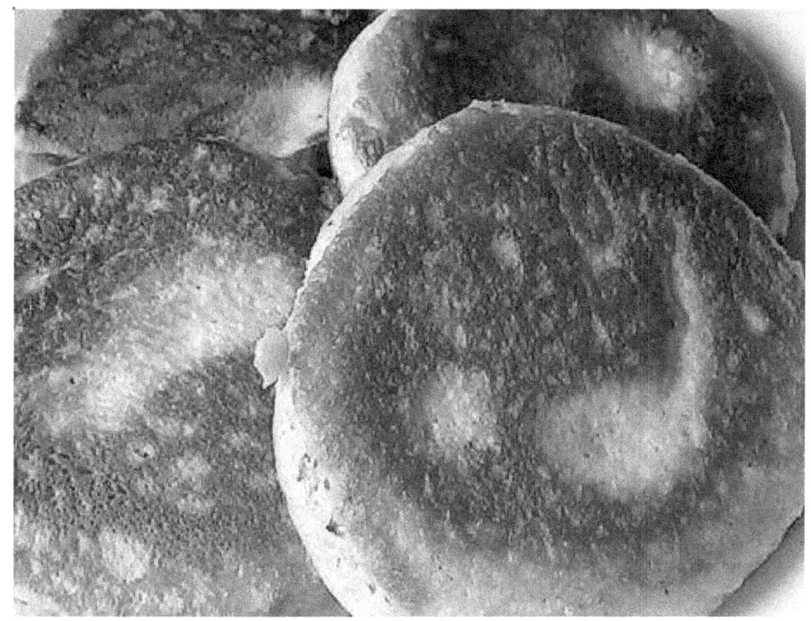

Ingredients for 1 portion

2	Egg
125 g	Hazelnuts, ground
5 ml	Sweetener, more fluid
2 tbsp.	Flour or egg white powder
1 tsp.	ground cinnamon
	Whole milk, 3.5% fat

1 pinch salt

Oil, for frying

Possibly.   Cinnamon powder, to sprinkle

Preparation

Total time approx. 30 minutes

Place eggs, hazelnuts, sweeteners, flour, cinnamon, milk and salt in a mixing bowl and mix well with an electric hand mixer. The amount of milk should be chosen so that a viscous, but not too firm "porridge" arises. Put a ladle full of dough into a hot, oil-frying pan and fry the pancakes until golden brown on both sides, making sure that the temperature of the pan is not too high.

Sprinkle the finished pancakes with cinnamon as desired.

Tip: If you want to further reduce the carbohydrates and increase the protein content, you can also use some protein powder instead of the flour.

FIG DESSERT

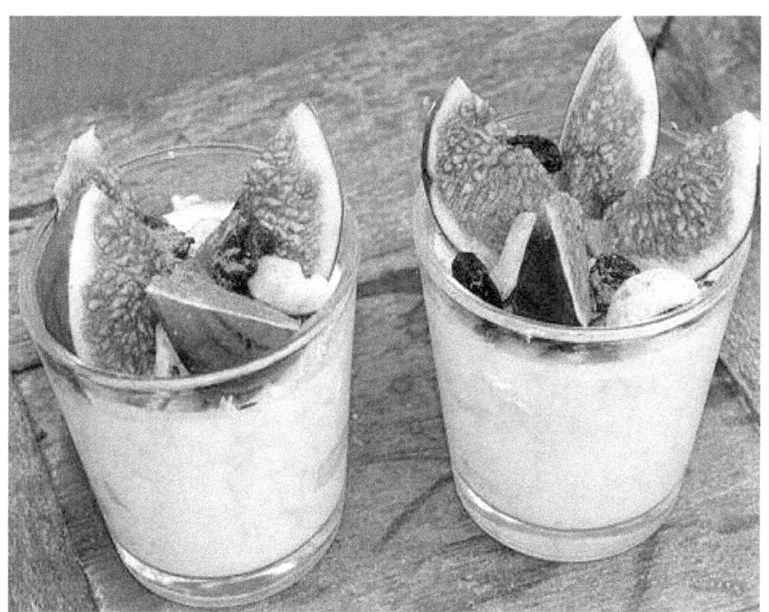

Ingredients for 1 portion

1 big   Fig

1 cup   Natural yoghurt

3 tsp. heaped   Muesli (Crunchy Muesli)

          Agave nectar

Some   cashews

1 tbsp.   Cranberries

          Cinnamon

Preparation

Total time approx. 6 minutes

Put the yoghurt in a bowl. Wash the fig, remove the stalk and cut the fruit;

Layer the crunchy cereal over the yoghurt and drape the fig pieces on top. Distribute the cashews between the fig pieces, sprinkle with cranberries, drizzle the agave syrup over them and finally sprinkle the dessert with cinnamon.

LOW CARB WAFFLES

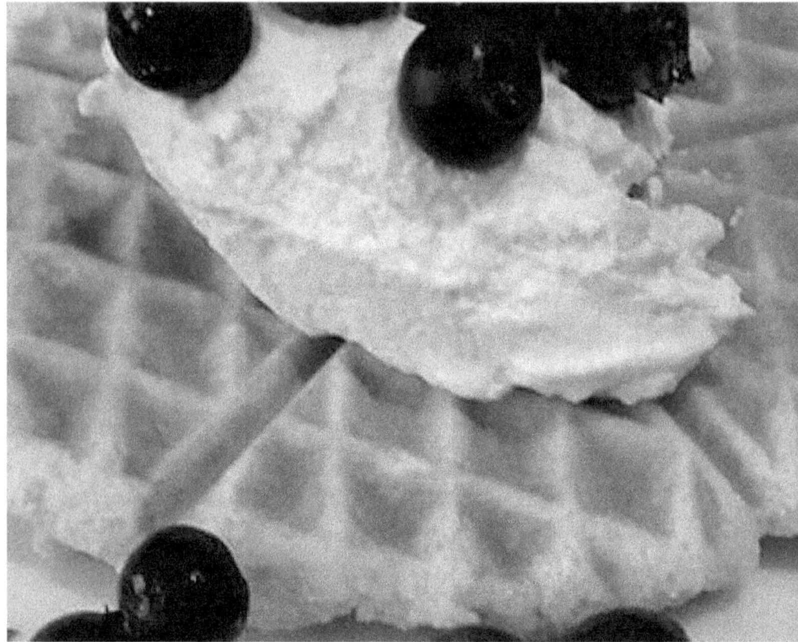

Ingredients for 1 portion

3   Egg

1 tbsp. Xylitol (sugar replacement)

1 pinch salt

2 tbsp.   Butter, melted

¼ tsp.   baking powder

50 g   coconut flour

Preparation

Total time approx. 20 minutes

Beat the eggs with sugar and salt until frothy. Mix the baking powder and coconut flour together and fold them in with the melted butter.

Bake the waffle batter as usual in a greased waffle iron.

LOW CARB DESSERT

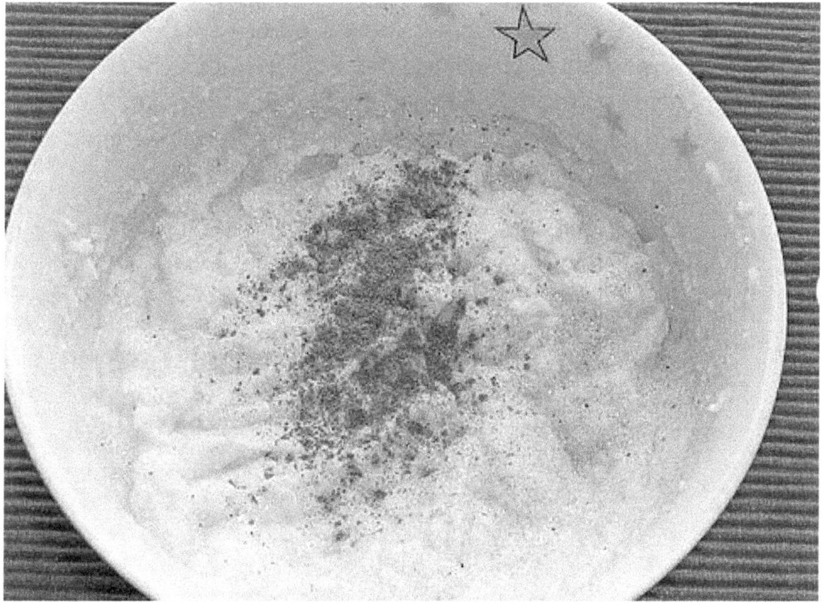

Ingredients for 2 portions

500 g   cauliflower

¾ package   Cream cheese (be careful: reduced fat often reduces the taste)

1 tsp.   Sweetener, (stevia or other sweetness at will)

1 teaspoon   Lemon zest or orange peel, finely grated

Preparation

Total time approx. 15 minutes

The origin of this recipe is a hearty low carb puree, which thanks to the relatively tasteless cauliflower can also be wonderfully sweet prepared. This dish is best compared with semolina pudding, but it is still a very special taste and thanks to the cream cheese also a touch of salty.

Boil the cabbage, depending on the desired consistency slightly bite or softer. As soon as it is cooked, puree with the cream cheese, also here you can use more or less cream cheese depending on the desired consistency of the porridge. Then sweeten the porridge with stevia or the desired sweetener, add the citrus peel, stir well and chill the porridge.

DELICIOUS LOW CARB QUARK DESSERT

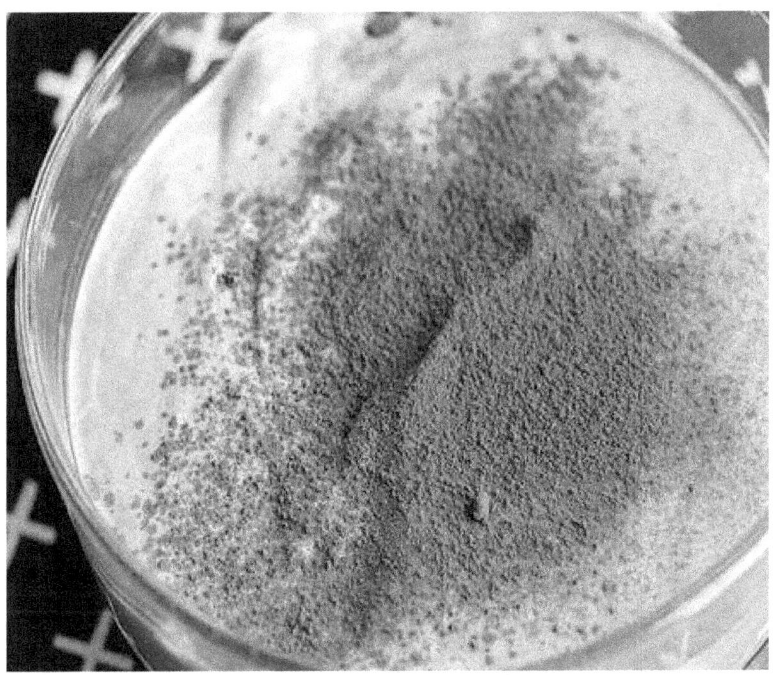

Ingredients for 1 portion

1 pck.   low-fat quark

2 tbsp. water

2 tbsp. Cocoa powder, de-oiled and unsweetened

2 Tea spoons   Sweetener, liquid, less as needed

          Vanilla flavor or orange flavor, liquid, sugar-free

Preparation

Total time approx. 5 minutes

Mix the curd cheese with water, sweetener and flavor until smooth and add the cocoa. Mix everything to a homogeneous mass.

FAST LOW CARB CHOCOLATE PUDDING

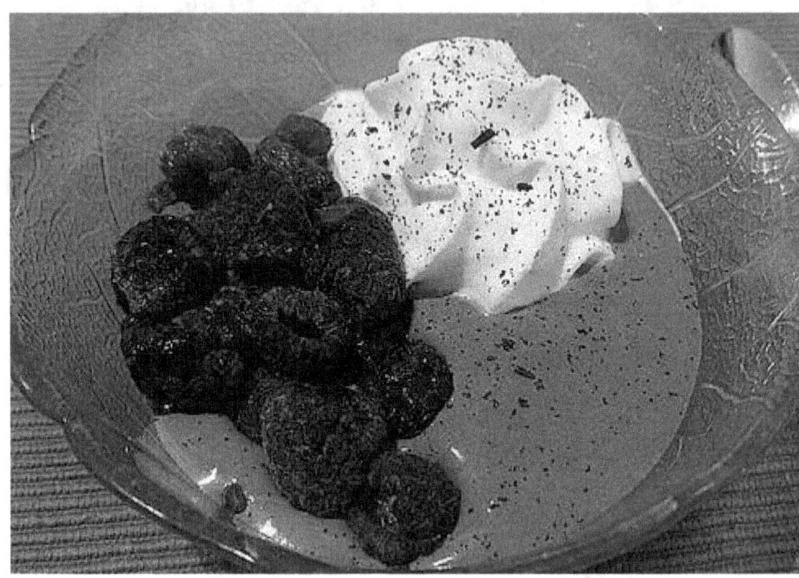

Ingredients for 2 portions

4 tsp.   cocoa powder

          Cream (whipped cream)

1 pck.   QimiQ classic

          Sweetener

Preparation

Total time approx. 40 minutes

Sift the baking cocoa into a small bowl and add as much cream (or milk if you want to save calories) until you get a thick cream that still flows from the spoon.

Stir the Qimiq creamy in a separate bowl and mix with the thick cocoa until no more lumps are visible. Season with sweetener. I have two splashes, then it is still strong chocolaty and not too sweet.

Either you can eat the pudding immediately, then it is of the consistency like cream pudding, or put in the fridge for about half an hour, then it solidifies a bit more.

LOW CARB TIRAMISU

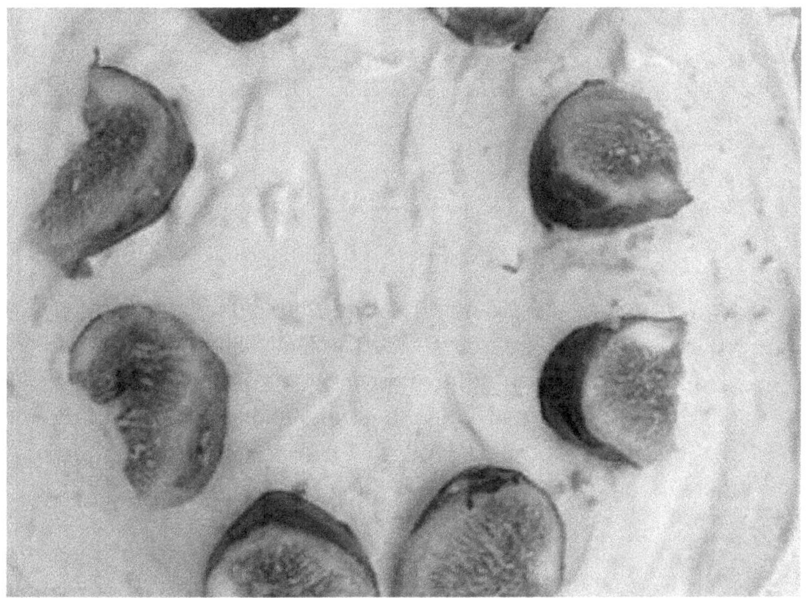

Ingredients for 1 portion

For the dough: (biscuits)

4   Egg

70 g   Xylitol (sugar replacement)

½ TL   baking powder

40 g   almond flour

For the cream:

500 g   mascarpone

250 g   Quark 20% or 40%

125 g   Powdered sugar from xylitol

7 tbsp. Amaretto, alternatively Amaretto

2   Espresso, strong

Cocoa powder for sprinkling

Preparation

Total time approx. 1 hour 42 minutes

For the biscuits, preheat the oven to 175 ° C (top / bottom heat).

Separate the eggs and beat the egg whites until stiff. Beat egg yolks and sugar until foamy, add the almond flour and carefully fold in the egg whites. Place the dough either in a freezer bag, cut off the corner and squirt the dough in portions onto the plate or simply form small piles with 1 - 2 tablespoons of dough. Bake in the oven for 10 - 12 minutes, then allow to cool briefly.

For the cream:

Mix mascarpone, quark, sugar and about 5 tablespoons Amaretto into a mixture. Possibly. a dash of milk if the mass is too firm.

In a bowl, mix the cold espresso with 2 tablespoons Amaretto.

Layer a layer of biscuits in a baking dish and add the mixture of espresso and amaretto, then cover with a layer of mascarpone mixture. Then another layer of biscuits, soak again with the espresso-Amaretto mixture. Finally, add the remainder of the mixture and sprinkle with cocoa powder.

Then put the finished Tiramisu at least for 1, better 2 - 3 h in the refrigerator.

LOW CARB PROTEIN ICE CREAM YOGURT & CHERRY

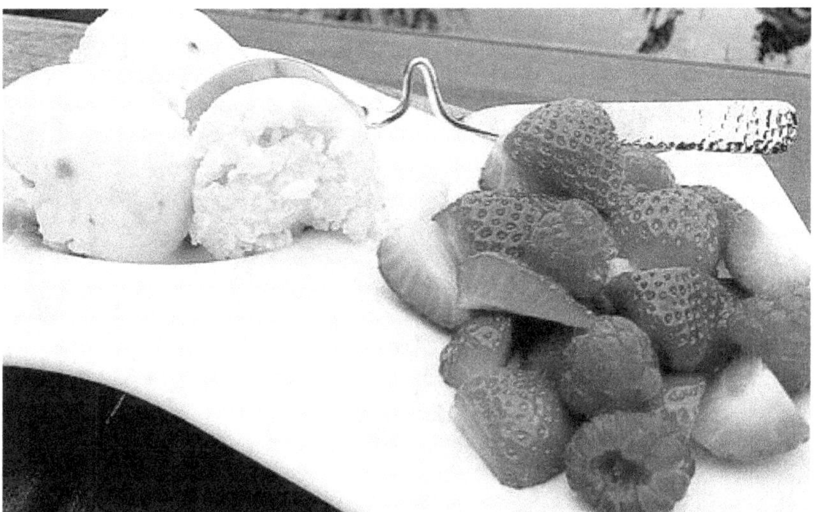

Ingredients for 3 portions

500 ml buttermilk

30 g   Protein powder (yoghurt & cherry flavor)

            Sweetener

Possibly.   Fruits for garnish

Preparation

Total time approx. 35 minutes

Mix all ingredients and then for 20 - 30 min. fill in the ice maker. If you like, you can then garnish the ice cream with fruit.

LOW CARB PANNA COTTA WITH STRAWBERRY SAUCE

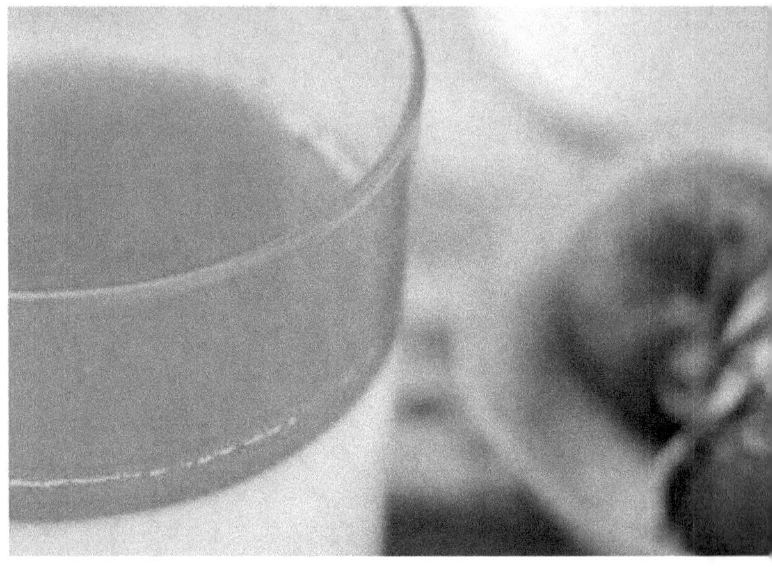

Ingredients for 4 portions

5 sheets   gelatin

600 ml whipped cream

1   Vanilla pod

120 g   strawberries

105 g   Xylitol (sugar replacement)

50 ml   water

Preparation

Total time approx. 4 hours 40 minutes

Soak the gelatin leaves in cold water as prescribed. Put the 600 ml cream with 70 g xylitol in a small saucepan and boil together. Press out the gelatin and put it in the saucepan. Stir gently until it dissolves. Meanwhile, scrape out the vanilla pod and put the pith in the hot cream.

Now provide a bowl of ice water. Put the still warm Panna Cotta out of the pot into a second bowl. Put these again in the bowl with the ice water. This is how the mass cools down. Once the mass starts to gel and gets creamier, fill in the dessert glasses. This process prevents the vanilla from settling to the bottom

Cook the dessert glasses in the refrigerator for approx. 4 hours. Meanwhile, you can prepare the strawberry sauce. Wash the strawberries, dry, quarter and place in a saucepan. Add the remaining 35 g of xylitol and the 50 ml of water and bring to the boil. Then the easiest way to puree with a blender or blender.

Continue cooking for about 5-10 minutes until the desired consistency is achieved. Then brush the strawberry sauce through a sieve. Now put in a glass, or a sealable container and also let cool.

Serve with the Panna Cotta

LOW CARB COOKIE DOUGH

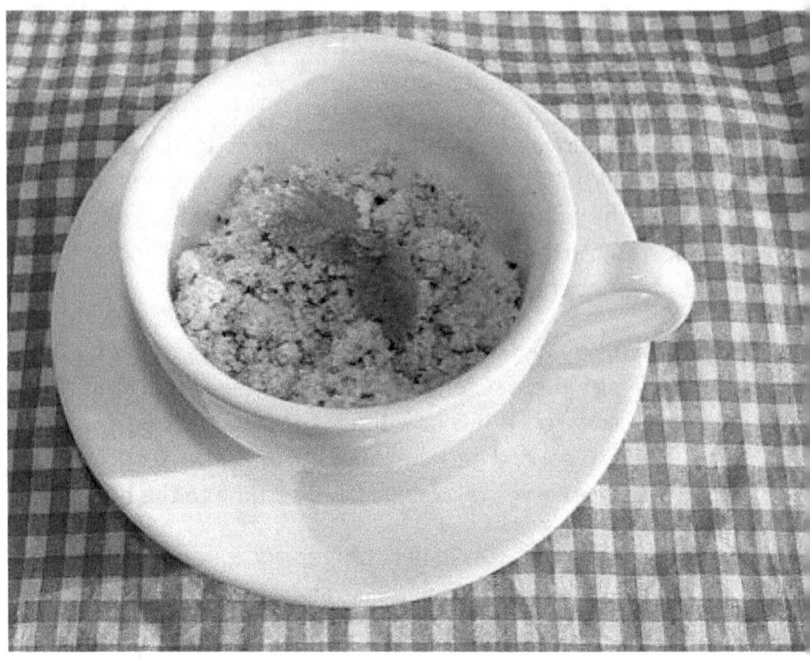

ingredients For 4 portions

120 g   almond flour

30 g   coconut flour

150 g   butter

80 g   Erythritol (sugar replacement)

120 ml milk

85 g   Chocolate drops without sugar

1 g   cinnamon

1 g   salt

10 drops   Aroma (cookie flavor)

Preparation

Total time approx. 10 minutes

Melt butter (microwave - low wattage).

Mix dry ingredients in a bowl.

Add 10 drops of cookie flavor to the liquid butter. Mix butter and milk with the dry ingredients. Add the chocolate drops to the dough.

Note: Instead of chocolate drops, of course, sugar-free chocolate can also be used. However, this must be hacked in advance.

CHOCOLATE CURD CASSEROLE LOW CARB

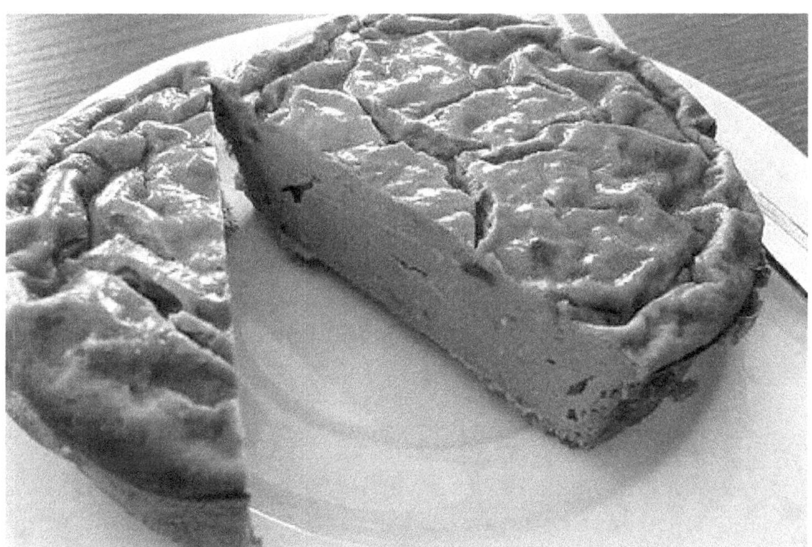

Ingredients for 1 portion

100 g   Cream cheese, grainy, light

100 g   low-fat quark

1 small   Egg

½ Pck.   Chocolate pudding powder

5 tbsp.   liquid sweetener

          Fruit of your choice

Preparation

Total time approx. 55 minutes

Mix all ingredients together. Add fruit at will.

Fill the mass into a baking dish and bake in a preheated oven at
approx. 190 ° C (top / bottom heat) for approx. 30 - 35 minutes.
Allow to cool for 15 minutes and serve.

HEARTY COFFEE CREAM, VEGAN AND LOW CARB

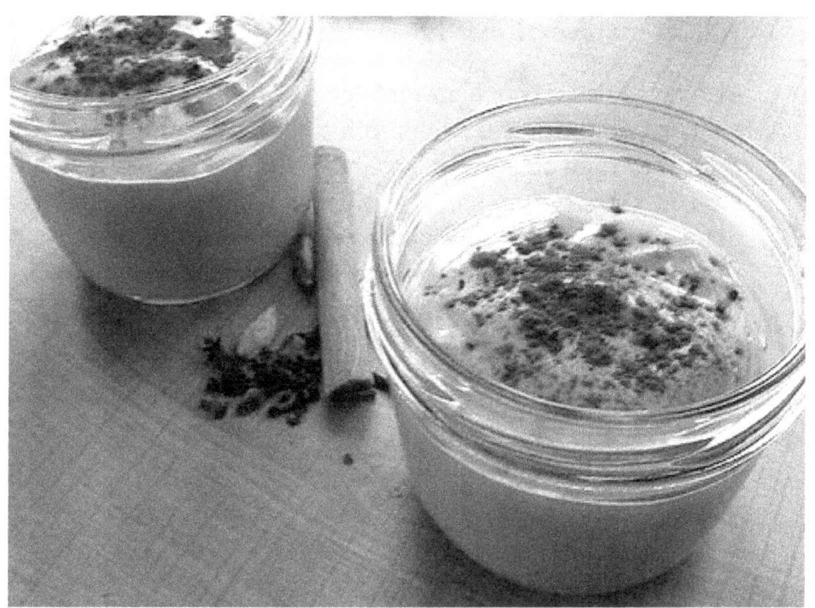

Ingredients for 2 portions

4 tbsp. Soy milk (soy drink)

3 tbsp. Coffee powder, instant

45 g   Sweetener with stevia

300 g   Soy quark (quark alternative), unsweetened

2 Tea spoons   ground cinnamon

1 tsp.   cardamom powder

1 tsp.   ground cloves

1 teaspoon   vanilla

         Cocoa powder, unsweetened

         Soy Cream (Soy Cream Cuisine)

Preparation

Total time approx. 2 hours 20 minutes

Mix the soy milk, coffee powder and sweetcorn together and heat at medium heat until the coffee powder is completely dissolved. Then pour into a large bowl and fold in the soybean curd. Mix the mixture thoroughly until a homogeneous mass is obtained. Now, gradually add cinnamon, vanilla, cardamom and clove powder and season to taste. Stir well again and refrigerate for at least 2 hours.

Garnish with unsweetened cocoa powder and soy cream as desired.

Tip: This will fit in the Christmas time homemade low carb cookies.

LOW CARB CINNAMON ROLL WITH GREEK YOGHURT

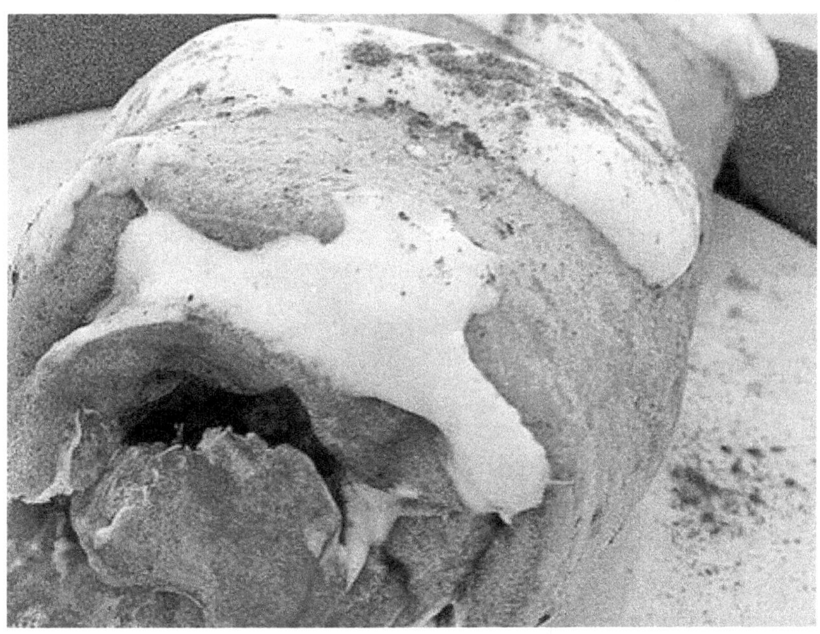

Ingredients for 1 portion

3   protein

1   Egg

2 tbsp. Powder, (protein powder), taste at will

30 g   Almond, grated or almond flour

1 teaspoon   baking powder

1 teaspoon   vanilla powder

60 ml   Almond milk (almond drink), or soy milk

1 tbsp. ground cinnamon

120 ml Yogurt, Greek

Stevia

Preparation

Total time approx. 30 minutes

Preheat the oven to 250 degrees. Mix egg whites, egg, protein powder, grated almonds or almond flour, baking powder, vanilla, almond or soy milk and cinnamon. If you like it sweet, you can add a dash of sweetener or stevia.

Lay out a round spring form pan with baking paper. Fill in the dough and smooth it out. Bake for 10 minutes.

Remove from the mold, brush with yoghurt and roll up. Fix it with a skewer. Garnish the roll with a little yoghurt and decorate with fruits or berries as desired.

LOW-CARB MINI CAKES WITH CHIA SEEDS AND BERRIES

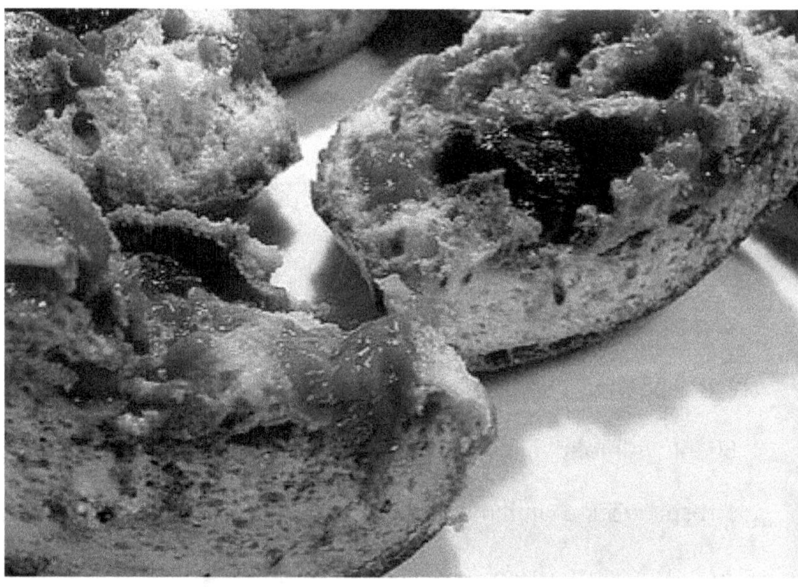

Ingredients for 2 portions

5 tbsp. Powder, (vanilla protein)

50 g   Berries

1 teaspoon   baking powder

2   Eggs

3 tbsp. Milk, low-fat

1 teaspoon   Stevia

1 tbsp. Seeds, (Chia-)

Preparation

Total time approx. 55 minutes

Separate the eggs and beat the egg whites until stiff. Preheat the oven to 200 degrees.

In a bowl, mix the protein powder, the baking powder and the milk. Add the egg yolk and carefully lift the egg whites underneath. Add stevia as needed.

Lift the chia seeds and the frozen berries under the mass. Pour the mixture into 2 small cake pans and bake in the oven for 35-40 minutes.

LOW CARB CHOCOLATE CREAM

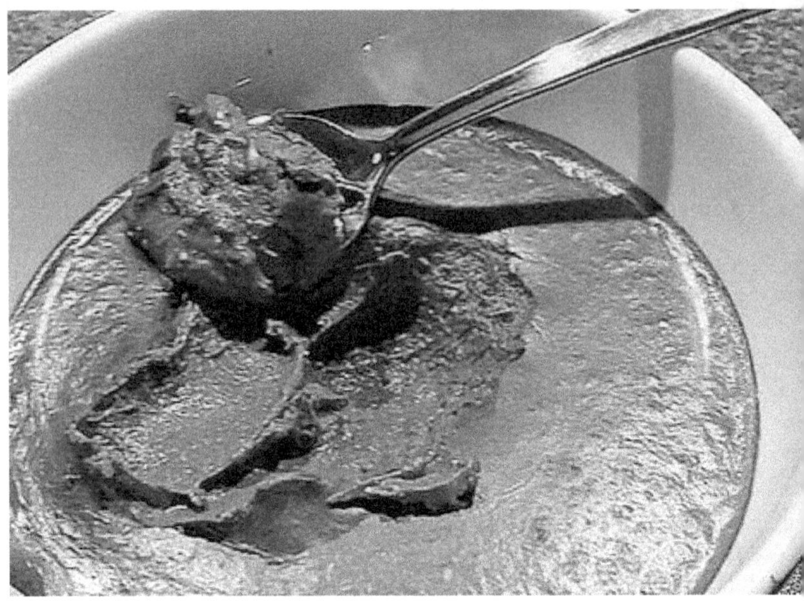

Ingredients For 4 portions

2 Large protein

1   egg yolk

500 g   low-fat quark

15 g   Cocoa powder, (baking cocoa)

100 ml milk

20 g   Almond, ground

5 splashes   sweetener

         Fruit, optional

Preparation

Total time approx. 15 minutes

Beat 2 egg whites until stiff. Separately mix the lean quark, milk, 1 egg yolk, ground almonds and the sweetener creamy. Then add the egg whites and sprinkle on the cocoa (for me it was about 15g - but you can also use more or less, depending on how chocolaty it should taste). Then mix the cocoa well with the remaining mass. The almonds are not a must, but make the cream firmer and tastier. If you want, you can add some fruit (strawberries are just fine). Then put in the fridge for about 1 hour.

LOW CARB APPLE PIE

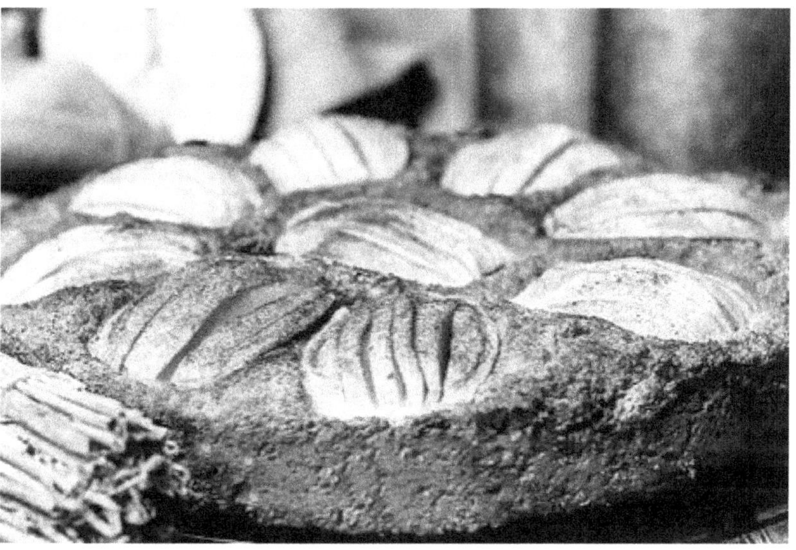

Ingredients for 1 portion

100 g   coconut flour

30 g   Walnut flour or hazelnut flour, de-oiled

5 g   Psyllium shell flour

15 g   potato fibers

120 g	Butter, room warm
6	Eggs
160 g	Xylitol (sugar replacement)
½ Pck.	baking powder
80 ml	Milk or coconut milk
3	apples
20 g	Xylitol (sugar replacement)

Preparation

Total time approx. 1 hour 25 minutes

Preheat oven to 175 ° C circulating air. Peel apples, remove core casing, cut into quarters and then fan in the quarters at the back. Whisk eggs and xylitol in a mixing bowl until frothy. Gradually add butter and beat until foamy.

In another bowl, mix coconut flour, nut flour, psyllium husk powder, potato fiber, baking powder and xylitol.

Grease a spring form with 26cm diameter with butter and powder with potato fibers.

Now carefully stir in the dry ingredients until a homogeneous dough is formed.

Now fill the dough in the Spring form and smooth it out. Spread apple pieces on the dough with the cut side up and lightly press.

Sprinkle the cinnamon-xylitol mixture over the cake. Bake at 175 ° C for 50 minutes. To serve, sprinkle with powdered xylitol.

LOW CARB RICE PUDDING

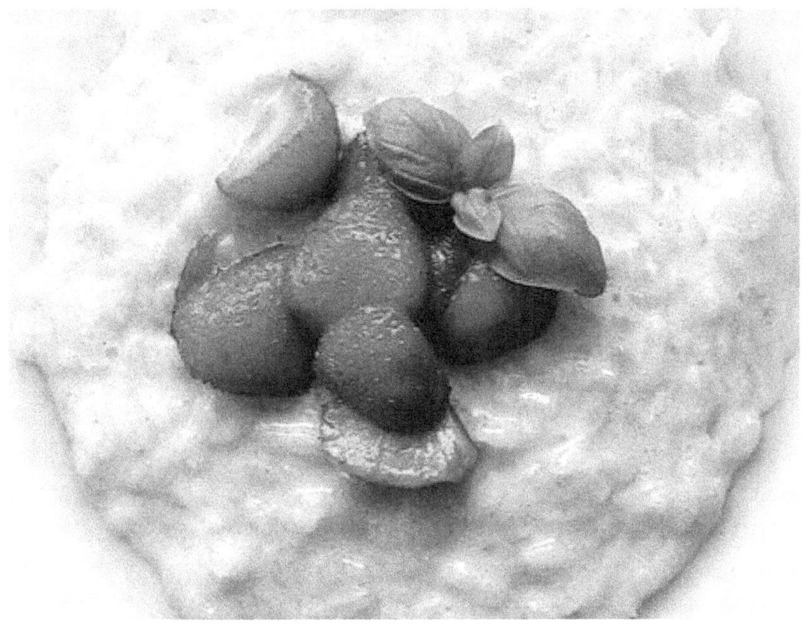

Ingredients for 1 portion

250 g   rice, drained

150 ml Milk or soy milk

½ tsp.   flour

2 tbsp. Honey or sweetener of your choice

½ tsp.   Vanilla pod, of which the marrow

½ tsp.   ground cinnamon

100 g   Fruits of your choice

Preparation

Total time approx. 8 minutes

Remove the rice from the packaging, drain off the water and rinse in a strainer with clean water. The rice may have a slightly fishy odor that flies away. Otherwise it is tasteless and takes on the taste of the ingredients.

Mix the milk with the flour as binder with a whisk well. Put the rice and the milk mixture in a saucepan and simmer for about 3 minutes on medium heat until the desired consistency is achieved.

Add the boiled rice pudding and add the vanilla and cinnamon. Important: taste it!

Wash the fruits, chop them and serve with the rice.

LOW CARB ICE CREAM SANDWICH

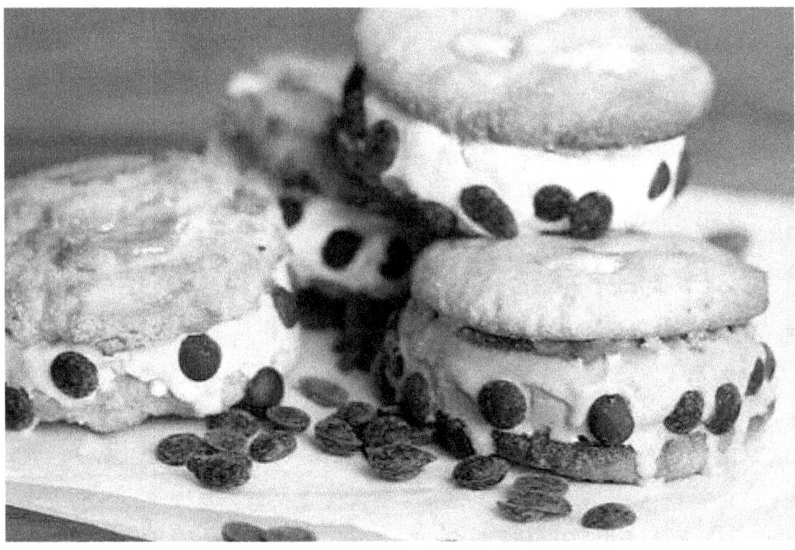

Ingredients for 3 portions

For the dough:

60 g	Xylitol (sugar replacement)
40 g	almond flour
2	egg yolk
1 tsp.	Xylitol (sugar substitute) (vanilla xylitol)
40 g	chokodrops (sugar-free, white chokodrops)

For the ice cream: (chocolate ice cream)

200 ml	Cream, struck stiff
1	egg yolk
30 g	Dark chocolate 80%
50 g	Xylitol (sugar replacement)

For the ice cream: (vanilla ice cream)

500 ml	Cream, struck stiff
5	egg yolk
2	Vanilla pod
150 g	Xylitol (sugar replacement)

For the ice cream: (coconut ice cream)

200 ml	Cream, struck stiff
150 g	coconut cream
50 g	Xylitol (sugar replacement)
30 g	Xylitol (sugar replacement)

Preparation

Total time approx. 6 hours 10 minutes

For the cookies, preheat the oven to 160 ° C, then mix all the ingredients for the dough, then stir in 2/3 of the chocolate drops.

Lay out a baking sheet with parchment paper. Divide the dough into 6 equal portions and shape small balls, then place on the plate and press flat. Then distribute the remaining chocolate drops on the cookies. Bake cookies for 12 minutes at 160 ° C convection. Then let cool down, otherwise they will break.

Then prepare one or more ice creams of your choice, here chocolate, vanilla or coconut ice cream.

Chocolate ice cream: put on a water bath. Melting chocolate over the water bath. Stir in xylitol and egg yolk.

Whip the cream. Mix 1 - 2 tablespoons of the whipped cream under the chocolate mixture, the chocolate cools down a bit, but does not clot. Then add the egg chocolate gradually to the stiff cream and stir until it gives a homogeneous mass. Place in the freezer for at least 6 hours (close well) and stir every 90 minutes.

Vanilla ice cream:

Whip cream until stiff. Place water bath. Put the yolks together with the xylitol in the bowl for the water bath. Scrape out the vanilla pods and add to the egg mass. Beat the egg mass over the water bath. Gradually add the egg mixture to the stiff cream and stir until it becomes a homogeneous mass. For at least 6 hours, place in the freezer (close well) and stir every 90 minutes.

Coconut ice cream: fry the

Coconut flakes with 30 g xylitol in the pan, taking care not to burn anything, then place in the refrigerator so that the cream does not liquefy again during the ice reunification. Whip the cream. Open a can of coconut milk, do not shake it before! And skim off the thick coconut cream with a tablespoon. Then mix the coconut cream with the remaining xylitol. Lift under the stiff whipped cream. Now fold in the grated coconut and place in the container to freeze. Place in the freezer for at least 6 hours (close well) and stir once in a while. The risk of ice crystal formation is lower here by the coconut flakes.

After you put the ice in the freezer for 6 hours, you can start the ice cream sandwich production.

For this, you spread a cookie with a layer of ice, put a second cookie on top of it and smooth out any uneven spots with a knife. If you want, you can now decorate the rim with chocolate.

Now you can immediately enjoy your ice cream sandwiches or put them in stock in your freezer.

LOW CARB PROTEIN FLUFF WITH FRUIT

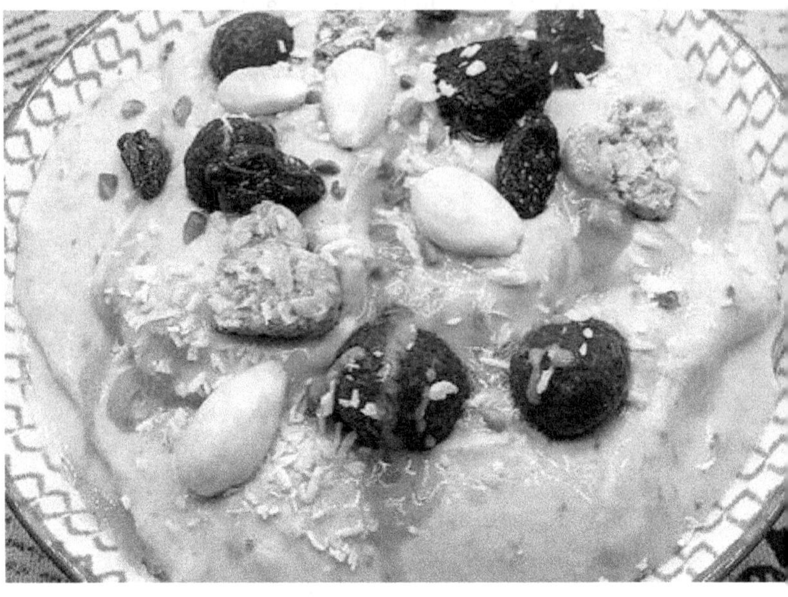

Ingredients For 1 portion

100 g   Fruits (Strawberries, raspberries, mango)

100 ml   Juice or water

1   protein

Stevia, sweetener, or similar

2 g   xanthan

Preparation

Total time approx. 5 minutes

Puree the frozen fruits with the liquid in the blender. Beat the egg whites until stiff.

Stir fruit with egg white, sweetener and xanthan cream for about 2 minutes with the hand mixer.

LOW CARB WAFFLES WITH BERRIES

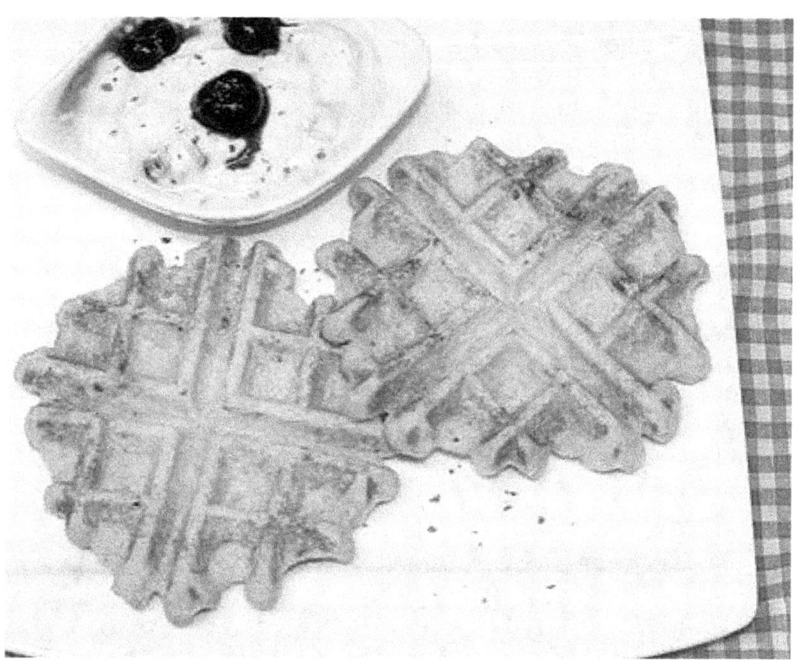

Ingredients for 2 portions

4   Egg

60 g   butter

100 g   Quark

2 tbsp. oil

6 tbsp. Protein powder with vanilla flavor

125 g   Berries, mixed

250 g   yogurt

Preparation

Total time approx. 40 minutes

Beat the eggs with butter (soft), cottage cheese and oil until foamy. Stir in the egg white powder. Bake the waffles one at a time in a hot, greased waffle iron and keep the waffles warm.

Lightly crush the berries and lift them loosely under the yoghurt. Serve waffles with berry yoghurt.

LOW-CARB COTTAGE CHEESE

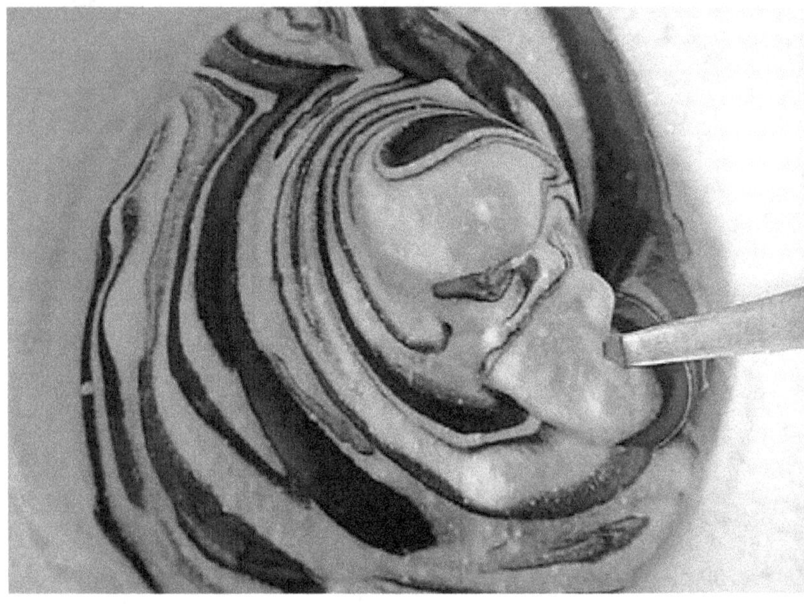

Ingredients for 1 portion

500 g   Quark, 20% fat

3 tbsp. cream

100 ml skimmed milk

2 tbsp. Nut nougat cream

Preparation

Total time approx. 5 minutes

Put the curd in a bowl. Stir in milk and cream well. Finally, add
the nut nougat cream and stir well.

The cream tastes like breakfast and a coffee snack. Since it is a
generous portion, you can divide this well. When buying the nut
nougat cream, make sure that as little carbohydrates and sugar
as possible are included.

TIRAMISU CREAM

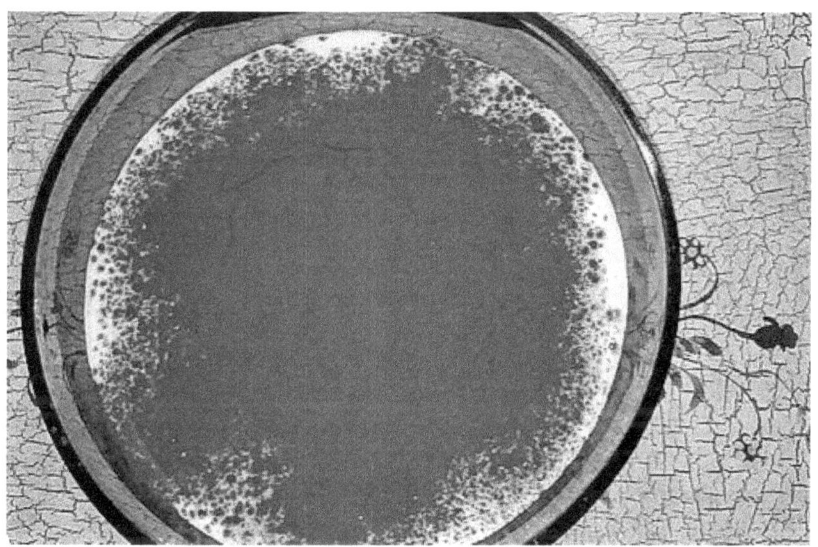

Ingredients for 2 portions

150 g   mascarpone

1   Egg

3 piece Sweetener, or Stevia tabs, best mixed for a rounder
sweetness

| 1 splash | rum |
| 1 teaspoon | cocoa powder |

Preparation

Total time approx. 7 minutes

Mix the mascarpone (about one-third of a 500 g beaker) with the egg yolk, the well-crushed sweetener tablets and a dash of rum until frothy. Then fold in the beaten egg whites. Fill in two bowls and sprinkle with cocoa powder.

HIGH-PROTEIN CLEANER SNICKERS QUARK

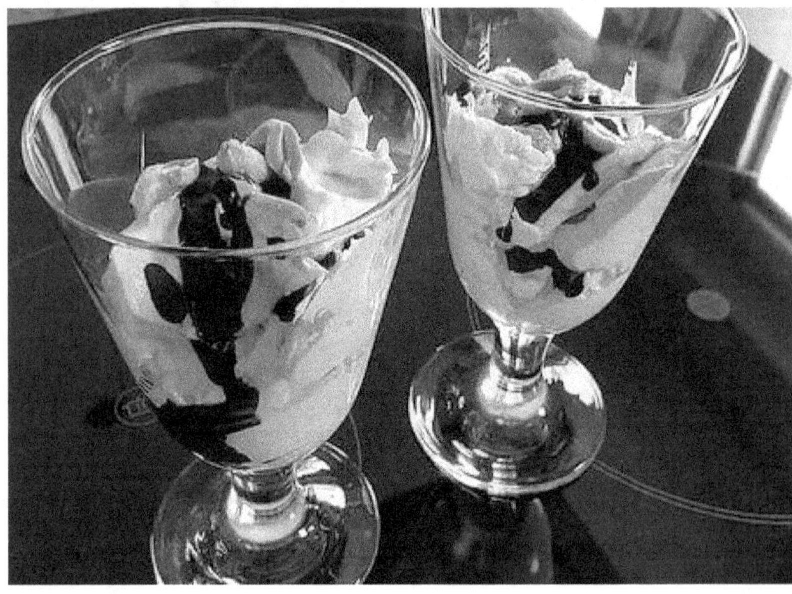

Ingredients for 1 portion

300 g   low-fat quark

10 g   peanuts

20 g	Peanut butter or peanut sauce
5 g	coconut oil
3 g	Back cocoa
5 g	Cornflakes or oat crunches
5 g	oatmeal
	Caramel syrup
	Schokodrops

Preparation

Total time approx. 10 minutes

Warm the coconut oil and mix with the peanuts, cocoa powder and oatmeal. Now mix the quark with the peanut butter. Then mix the cocoa mass with the quark.

Finally, decorate with oat crunches or cornflakes, peanuts and, if you like, chocolate drops and caramel syrup.

High in protein, low in carbohydrates and only good fats are included.

RASPBERRY QUARK WITH APPLE, FLAXSEED AND GOJI BERRIES

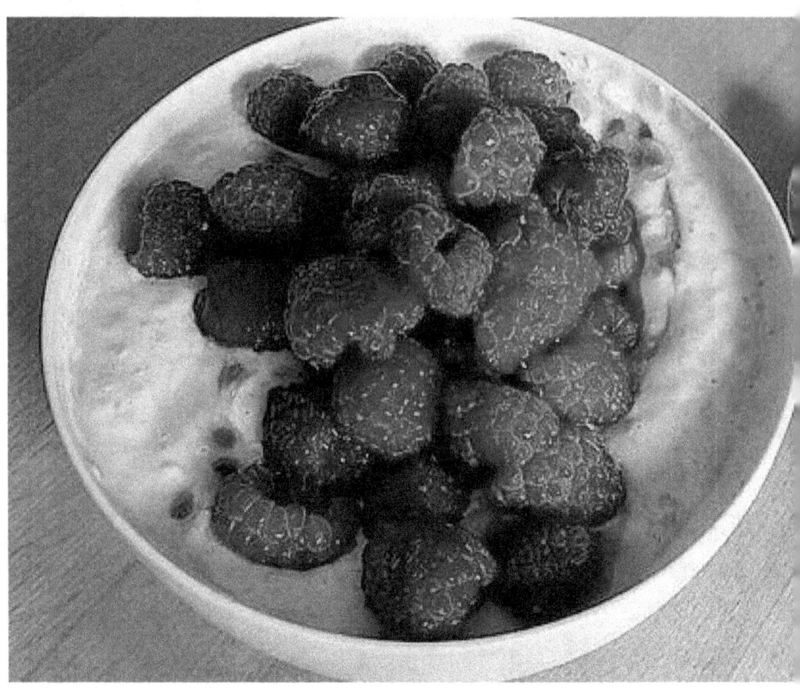

Ingredients for 1 portion

250 g   Quark, with 20% fat

150 g   Raspberries, thawed or fresh

2 tbsp.   milk

2 tbsp.   Applesauce, without sugar

1 tbsp.   Berries, dried (goji berries)

2 tbsp.   Linseed - shot

1   Apple

Sweetener, liquid, (stevia)

Preparation

Total time approx. 10 minutes

Mix all but the apple together until a homogeneous mass has formed. Remove the core of the apple and then cut the apple into fine pins. Lift these under the quark mixture - done!

MANDARIN DESSERT WITH CHOCOLATE CHIPS

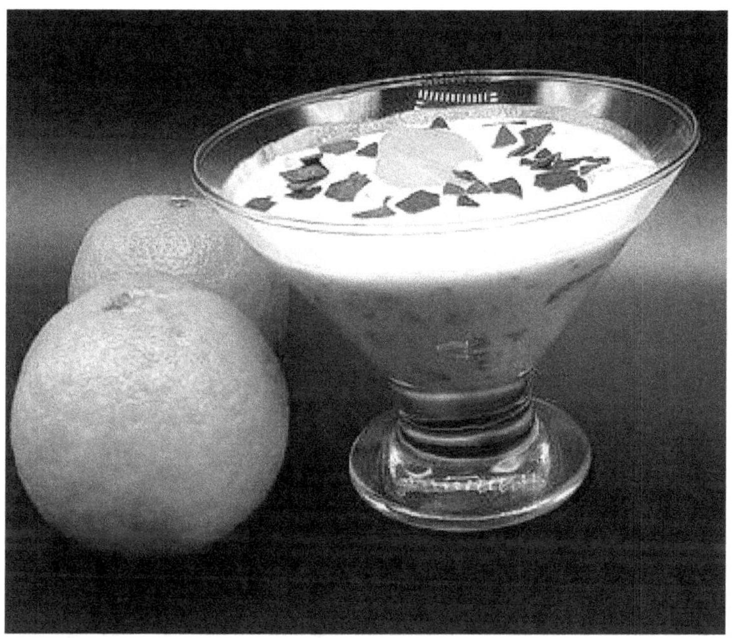

Ingredients for 6 portions

500 g   Quark, 20% (or 1x 40% and 1x 20%)

350 g   Yogurt, 3.5%

2   Tangerine, sweet

2 tbsp. Sugar, erythritol or xylitol, maybe more

2 tablespoons, heaped   chocolate, dark, grated

1 tsp.   cinnamon

Preparation

Total time approx. 10 minutes

Drain the tangerines well. Mix all other ingredients with the whisk. I always use self-grated 75 - 92% chocolate. Season the mixture and stir in the tangerines carefully.

CREAM CHEESE DESSERT WITH BERRIES

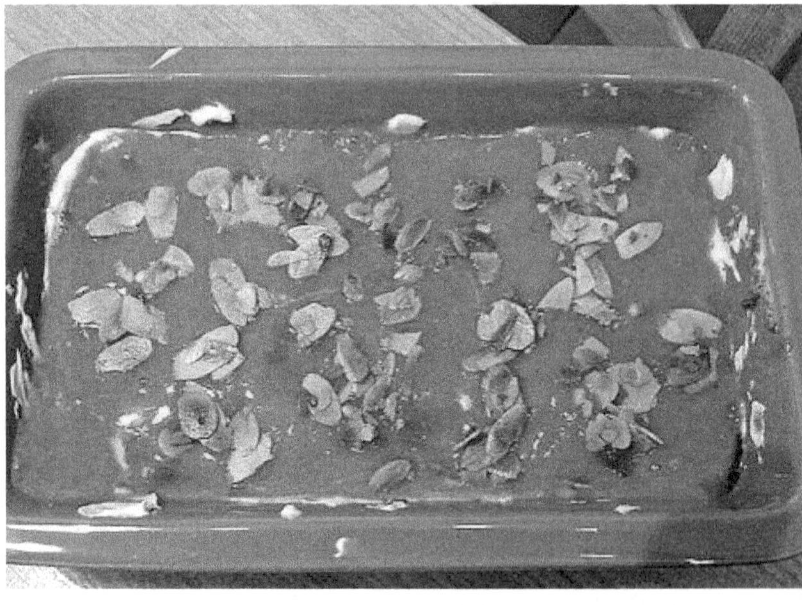

Ingredients for 6 portions

250 g   low-fat quark

250 g   cream cheese

200 g   whipped cream

5 ml   Sweetener, (replaces 100 g of sugar)

2 pck.   Sahnesteif

1 pinch Vanilla, (bourbon), freshly ground

1 pck.   Flaked almonds

250 g   Strawberries, or raspberries

Preparation

Total time approx. 1 hour 15 minutes

Roast the almond flakes golden brown and let cool. Watch out, they burn fast.

Beat the whipped cream with cream stiff. Mix the cottage cheese and cream cheese with the sweetener and vanilla in a bowl and fold in the whipped cream. Puree the berries. If you like, you can sweeten something.

You can either spread the cream on 6 glasses / dessert bowls or serve in a large bowl. Spread the berry sauce over the cream and chill until cold. Sprinkle the almonds just before eating to keep them crispy.

FAST RASPBERRY ICE CREAM

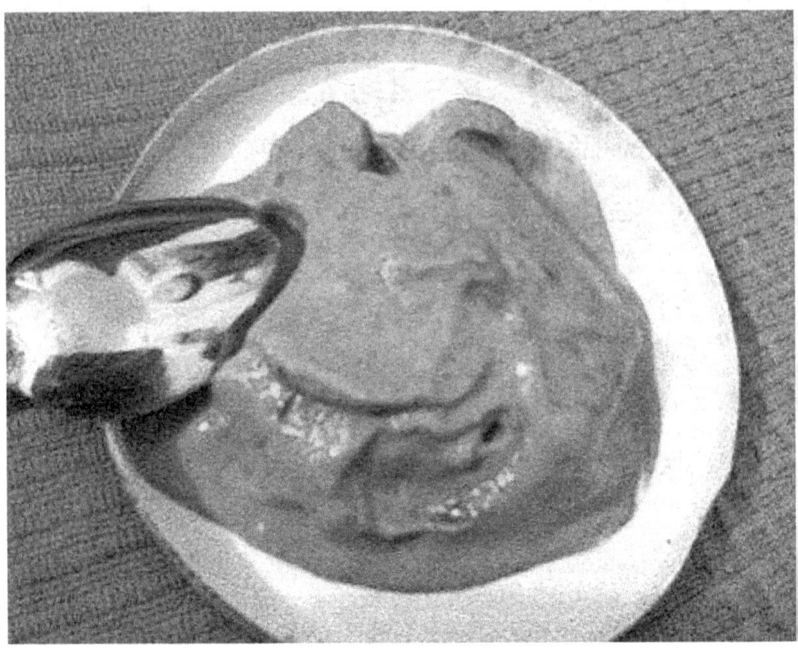

Ingredients For 2 portions

200 g   whipped cream

200 g   Raspberries, frozen, unsweetened

2 tbsp. Mandamus, white or brown

Preparation

Total time approx. 5 minutes

Put the cream in a tall container and stir in the almond paste. Then add the raspberries. The raspberries should come straight from the freezer and not be thawed yet! Carefully shred the raspberries with a hand blender and mix well.

The ice cream has a very creamy consistency and should be consumed immediately!

The almond paste can also be omitted, but it refines the taste
and improves the consistency.

QUARK CAM

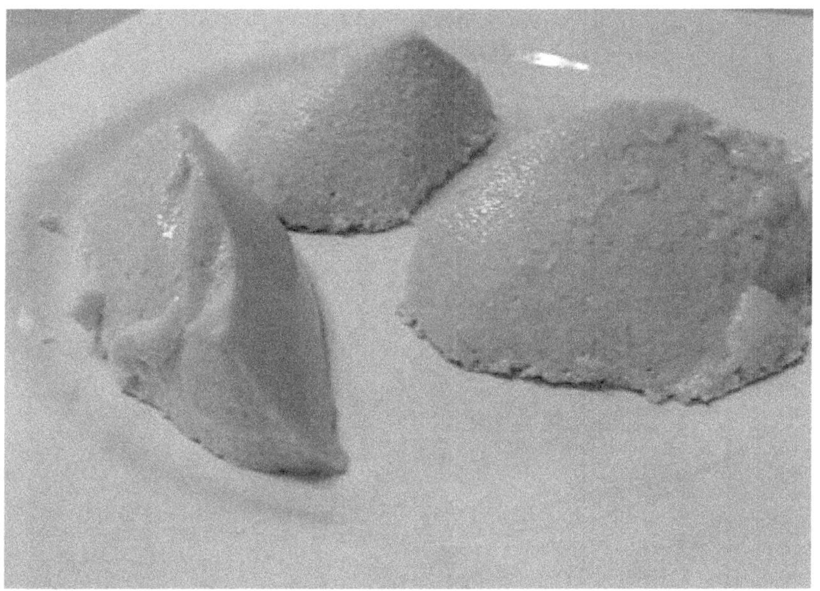

Ingredients for 4 portions

1 pck.   Jellies of your choice (lemon, cherry, woodruff)

500 g   low-fat quark

20 g   Protein powder of your choice (e.g. vanilla or coconut)

Liquid sweetener to taste

Preparation

Total time approx. 8 hours 5 minutes

Prepare the jellies according to instructions, replacing the sugar with sweetener. Gradually stir in the curd cheese, then add the protein powder to the mass.

Cold, preferably in the refrigerator overnight.

HIGH-PROTEIN CLEANER BOUNTY QUARK

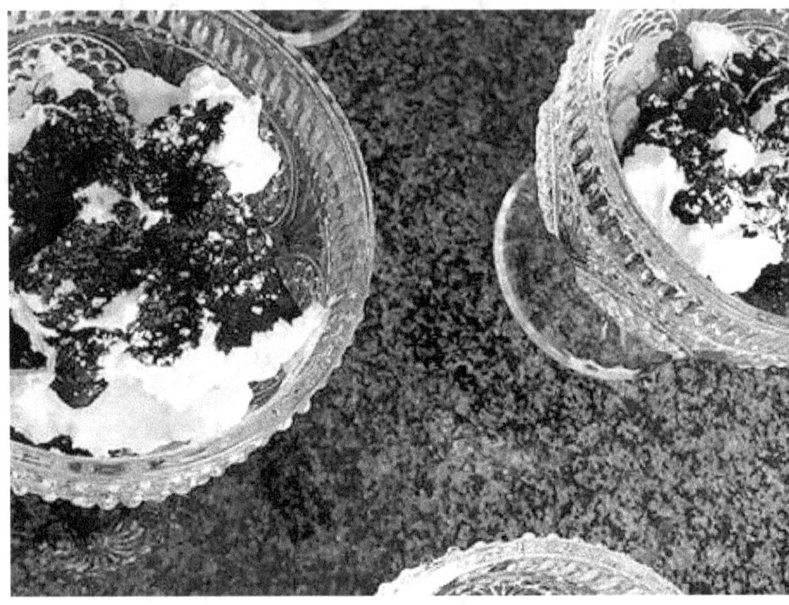

Ingredients for 1 portion

250 g   low-fat quark

1 tbsp. coconut oil

1 tbsp. Back cocoa

10 g   desiccated coconut

2 tbsp. Sugar or erythritol

Preparation

Total time approx. 40 minutes

Melt the coconut oil in the microwave. Mix with 1 tsp sugar or erythritol and 1 tbsp. cacao. Mix the quark with the remaining erythritol and a few coconut flakes.

When everything is well mixed, add some grated coconut under the liquid chocolate and stir again. Then pour the liquid cocoa chocolate over the quark and refrigerate everything in the fridge for about 30 minutes.

PARTY DESSERT

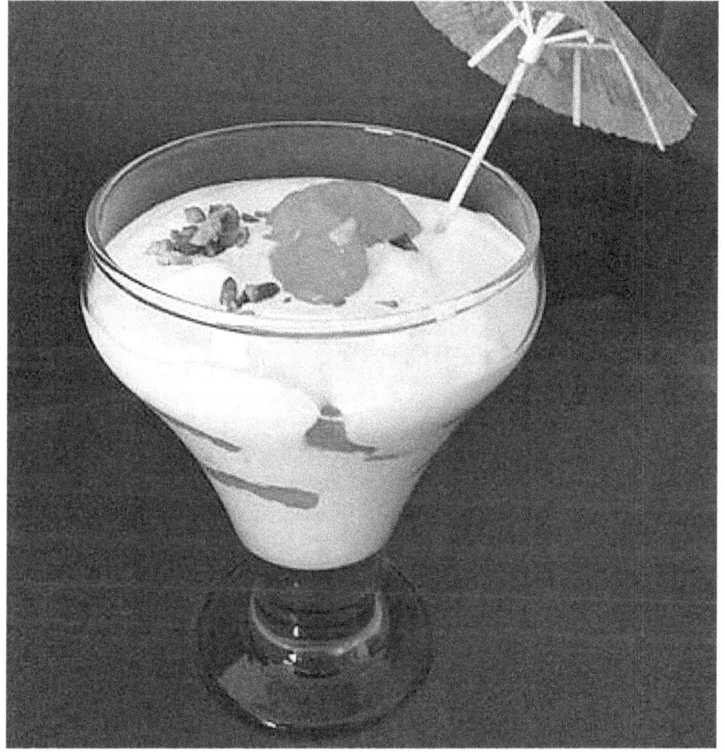

Ingredients for 10 portions

4 cups   sour cream

4 cups   whipped cream

4   Mandarin

10 pts   vanilla

4 pts.   Sahnesteif

Preparation

Total time approx. 10 minutes

Mix sour cream with vanilla sugar. Stir in the yoghurt and drained mandarins under the sour cream and finally fold in the whipped cream.

You can also prepare well the day before and then store in the fridge. Decorate e.g. with tangerines and chocolate rolls.

MANGO - QUARK - DESSERT WITH WALNUTS

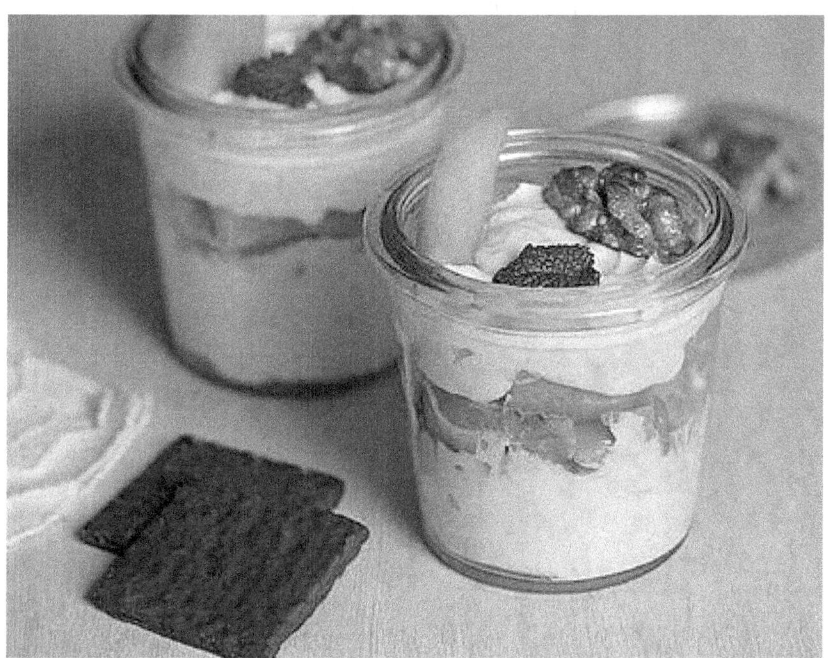

Ingredients for 8 portions

1 kg   Quark

200 g   cream

2 Large Mango, ripe

1   Lemon, untreated

1   Vanilla pod

50 g   walnuts

Sugar, at will.

Preparation

Total time approx. 15 minutes

Stir quark with the cream until smooth. Rub the lemon peel, squeeze out the lemon and put both into the quark. Cut the vanilla pod, scrape out the pith, chop the walnuts and add the quark with the vanilla pod. Peel mangos and cut into bite-sized cubes. Mix everything with the quark and sweeten to taste.

Cool before serving.

PLUM GRATIN WITH GOAT'S CHEESE

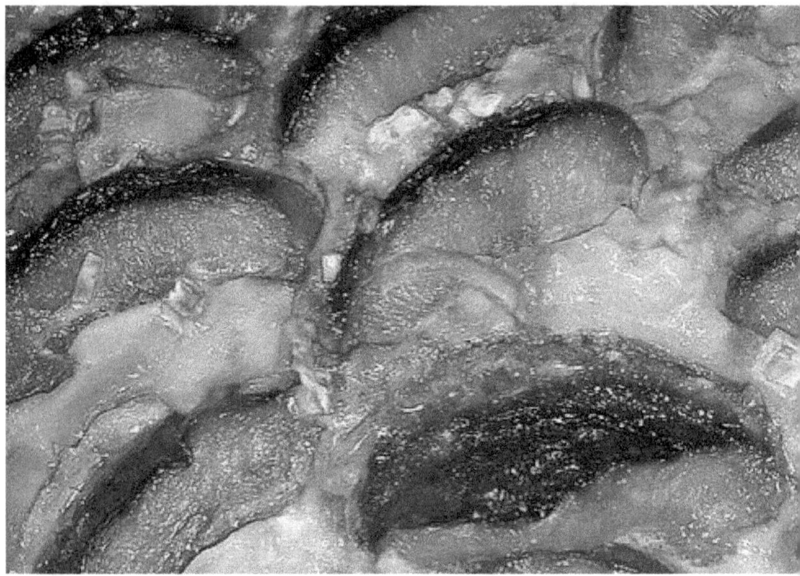

Ingredients For 4 portions

1 kg   Plum, ripe

2   Egg

100 ml cream

200 g   Goat cheese, (goat's cheese roll)

1   Vanilla pod, the marrow of it

1 pinch salt

Butter for greasing the mold

Preparation

Total time approx. 50 minutes

Wash, halve and stone so many prunes, dab them dry and place them in the buttered gratin / casserole dish, as if they fit into the mold. That can be 950 g, or 1050 g.

Beat the eggs until foamy, add the cream, vanilla pulp and the chopped goat's cheese with a pinch of salt and fold gently under the foam.

Pour this mixture evenly over the prunes into the mold (make sure that the cheese is "evenly distributed") and cook at 180 ° in the preheated oven for 20 minutes at bottom heat and then bake at 200 ° with bottom and top heat for 5 - 10 minutes until the surface gets color.

This gratin can be eaten hot, as is usual for a gratin, but I really prefer it cold, because the goat's cheese then tastes better and the other flavors harmonize better and you do not burn your mouth on the plums!

LOW CARB PROTEIN PANCAKES

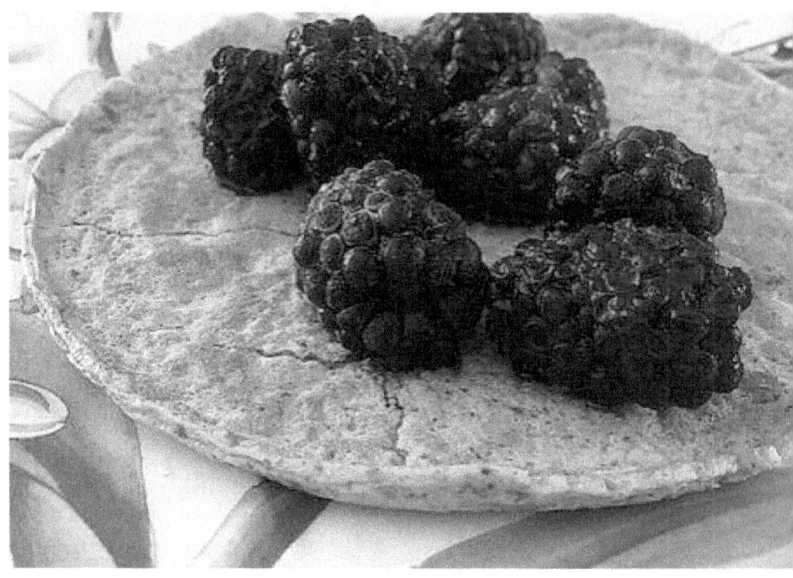

Ingredients for 1 portion

1 Large Egg

50 ml   Almond milk (almond drink), also coconut milk or cow's milk possible

7 tsp. heaped   Flax seed, crushed

Coconut milk, creamy

1 ½ tbsp.   protein powder

Preparation

Total time approx. 15 minutes

First, the egg is mixed with the almond milk and the creamy coconut milk to a homogeneous mass. Then simply add flaxseed to the blender and cut to the maximum level until it has the consistency of flour. Approximately 7 teaspoons of it and the protein powder (I have now taken Cookies and Cream) are now in the egg mixture.

Everything is stirred until a creamy consistency is obtained. Depending on how you want the mass, you can add some flaxseed flour or protein powder. The mass now comes in portions in the pan and is fried from both sides over medium heat.

LOW CARB GINGERBREAD CREME BRULEE

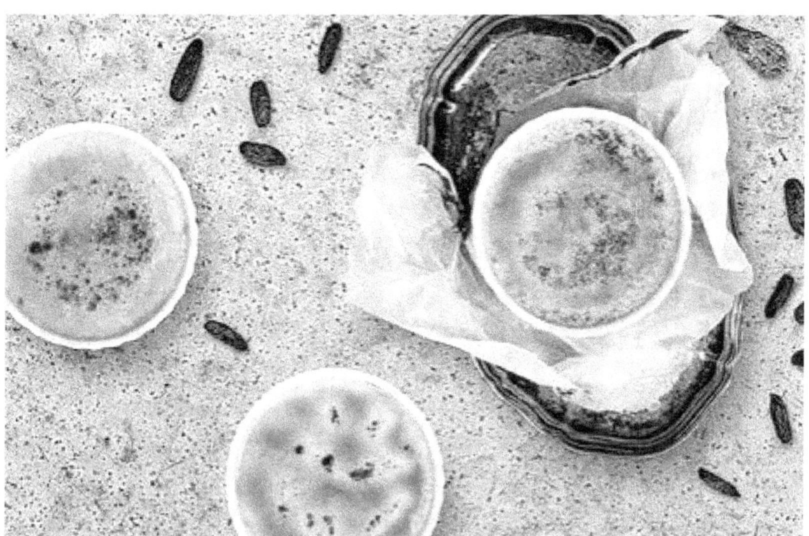

Ingredients for 4 portions

400 ml cream

75 g   Xylitol (sugar substitute) or erythritol

1 teaspoon   ginger bread spice

5   egg yolk

4 tsp   Erythritol (raw cane sugar substitute) for flambéing

Preparation

Total time approx. 1 hour 5 minutes

Preheat the oven to 125 ° C top and bottom heat.

Heat cream and xylitol in a saucepan. Add the gingerbread spice and bring the cream to a boil. Slowly stir the yolks into the cream mixture. Divide the crème Brule mixture into four ovenproof dishes and place in a casserole dish. Fill the casserole dish with water up to half of the cream bowls, place in the oven and let the cream falter for 50 minutes. Remove from the oven and let cool.

Sprinkle each bowl with 1 teaspoon brown sugar and flambé with a Bunsen burner, serve hot.

AVOCADO BANANA MOUSSE AU CHOCOLATE WITH PASSION FRUIT SAUCE

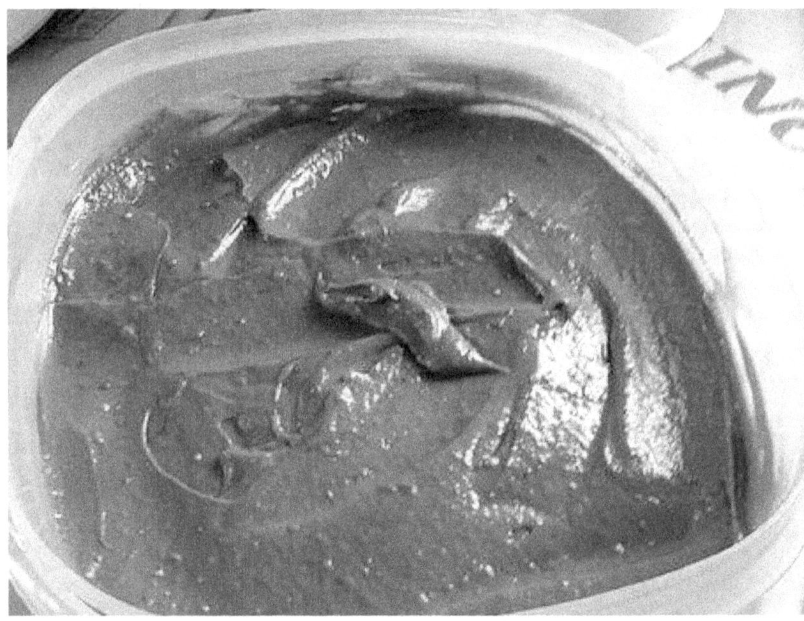

Ingredients for 4 portions

100 g   bitter chocolate

1   Avocado

1   Banana

100 ml whipped cream

2 tbsp. Grated chocolate, bittersweet

For the sauce:

4   Passion fruit

2 tbsp. agave syrup

Preparation

Total time approx. 2 hours 25 minutes

Melt the dark chocolate over the water bath and allow to cool. Puree avocado, banana and whipped cream, alternatively soy cream, etc. Stir in the melted chocolate. Put in glasses and refrigerate for 2 hours.

A fruit sauce tastes very delicious. Halve the passion fruits and scrape out the pulp. Boil with 2 tablespoons of agave syrup for 2 minutes and allow to cool.

To serve, sprinkle the mousse au chocolat with 2 tablespoons of dark chocolate grated chocolate and add the passion fruit sauce to taste or serve.

It also tastes great with other fruits, such as pureed strawberries.

CHIA ALMOND PUDDING WITH RASPBERRIES

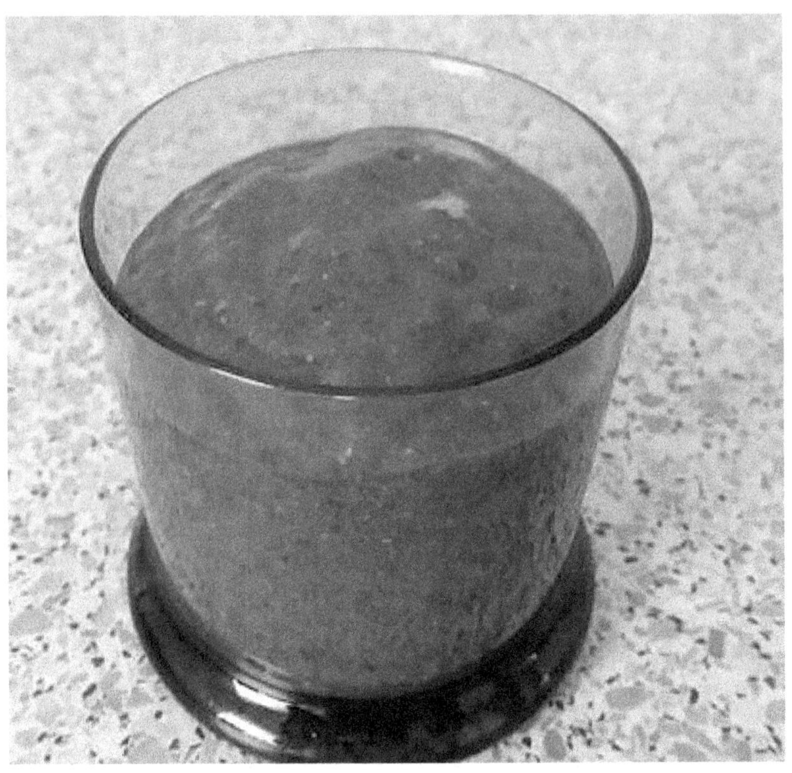

Ingredients for 1 portion

2 tablespoons, heaped   Chia seeds

200 ml Almond milk (almond drink), sweetened

125 g   raspberries

1 teaspoon   Xylitol (sugar replacement)

Preparation

Total time approx. 32 minutes

Stir the chia seeds into the almond milk. Approximately let it swell for 20 - 30 minutes, stirring once in between. Add sugar and raspberries and puree with the magic wand.

BEST LEMON CREAM ICE CREAM

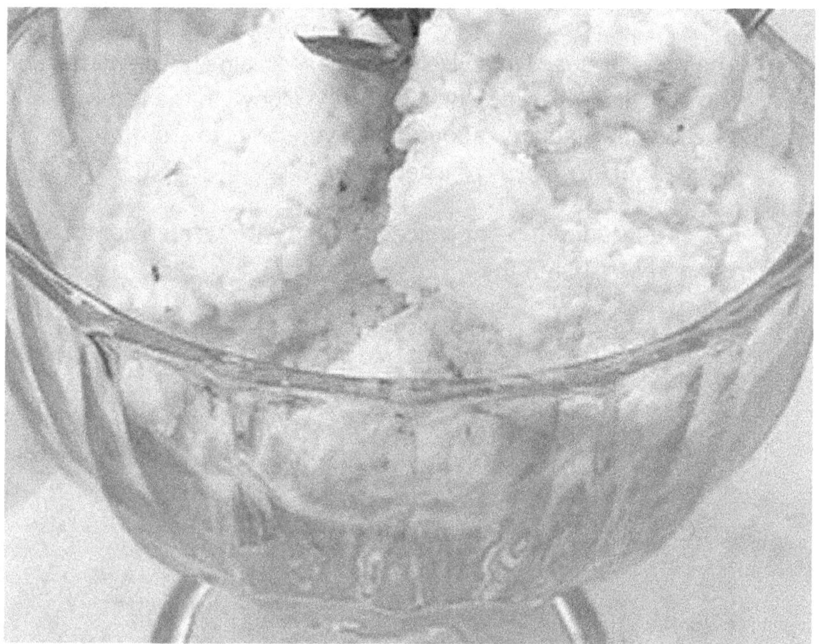

Ingredients for 4 portions

500 g   Skyr

2 small ones   Lemon, organic or untreated

4 splashes   Sweetener, liquid

10   Mint leaves, fresh

          Mineral water approx. 100 ml

Preparation

Total time approx. 5 minutes

Rub the lemon peel of both fruits with a grater and squeeze out the lemons. The sweetener, lemon juice and shells with a whisk with the Skyr mix. Finely chop the mint and fold in the same way. Mix the mass with a little mineral water (100 ml is sufficient) but do not whip up too much. The result should be homogeneous and similar in consistency to a pancake batter.

The mass either a) in an ice machine according to the manual of the device freeze with stirring or b) in a bowl in the icebox / freezer and regularly, about once every hour to stir until the desired consistency is reached.

The preparation time in an ice machine with its own compressor takes about 45 minutes.

LOW CARB GERM DUMPLINGS

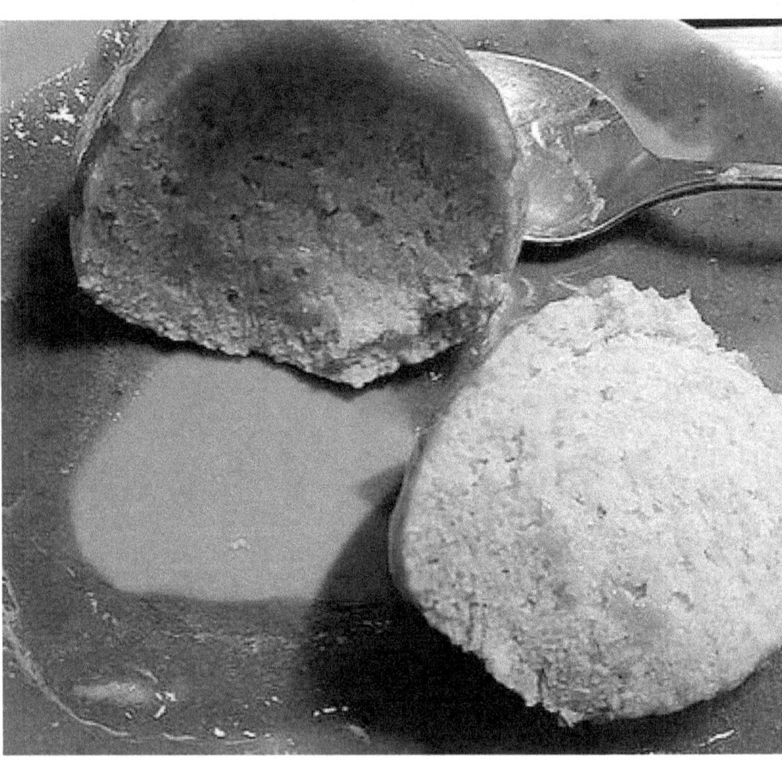

Ingredients for 4 portions

20 g   gluten

20 g   Psyllium husk, ground

60 g   oat bran

20 g   Protein powder (vanilla protein powder)

80 g   coconut flour

8 tbsp. Xylitol (sugar replacement)

1   Egg

1   protein

1 cube yeast

200 ml Milk with 0.3% fat

Preparation

Total time approx. 2 hours 30 minutes

Mix all dry ingredients in a mixing bowl. Dissolve the yeast in the lukewarm milk and add to the flour mixture. Add egg and egg whites and knead well. If the dough is too firm, add some milk. If it is too liquid, add some coconut flour. Who likes, can add other spices, such as vanilla, cinnamon or the like.

The dough should have the consistency of a standard dough and no longer stick to the edges of the bowl. Leave the dough in a warm place for at least 1 hour.

Divide the dough into 4 parts, shape them into balls and press flat. Optionally, you can add a filling, such. Jam, plum jam, poppy seed or pureed fruits. If you do without a filling, you can save on flattening and instead just form balls. Who fills the dumplings, should make sure that the dumplings are well closed, so that the filling does not leak during cooking. Cover the finished dumplings covered a bit.

Cook for about 20 - 25 minutes in a steamer or a steamer for the pot.

Serve warm with vanilla sauce or fruit compote.

VEGAN LOW CARB PROTEIN PANCAKES

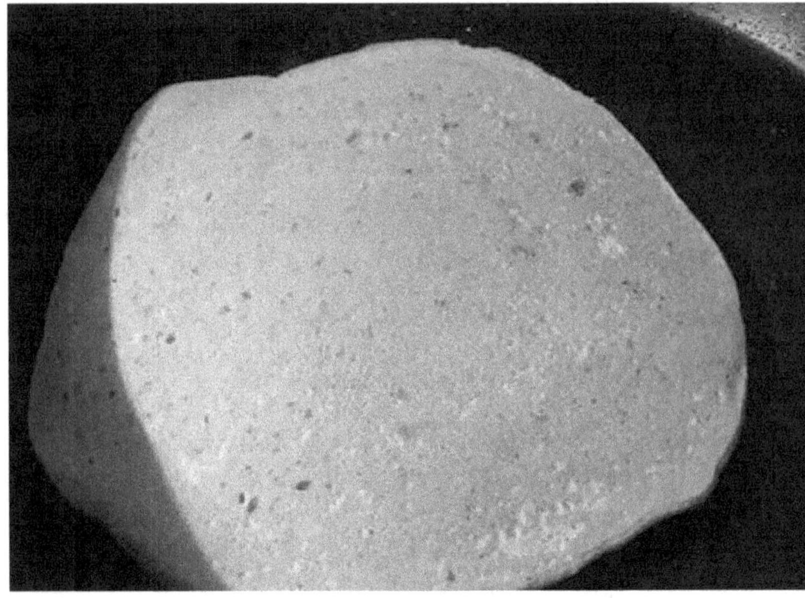

Ingredients for 2 portions

180 g   Wheat flour or spelled flour

120 g   Almond flour, white, de-oiled

520 ml Soy milk (soy drink)

3 tsp. heaped   protein powder

3 tbsp. Xylitol (sugar substitute) light or 2 tbsp. sugar

1 package   vanilla sugar

1 package   baking powder

1 tbsp. Apple Cider Vinegar

2 drops Taste of rum

1 pinch cinnamon

1   Banana, ripe or 3 tablespoons applesauce

Oil for frying

Preparation

Total time approx. 35 minutes

First mix all dry ingredients with a whisk. Then mix the wet ingredients separately for a short time and then add. Mix everything and fry in portions in a little oil in a pan.

LIGHT CHEESECAKE CREAM

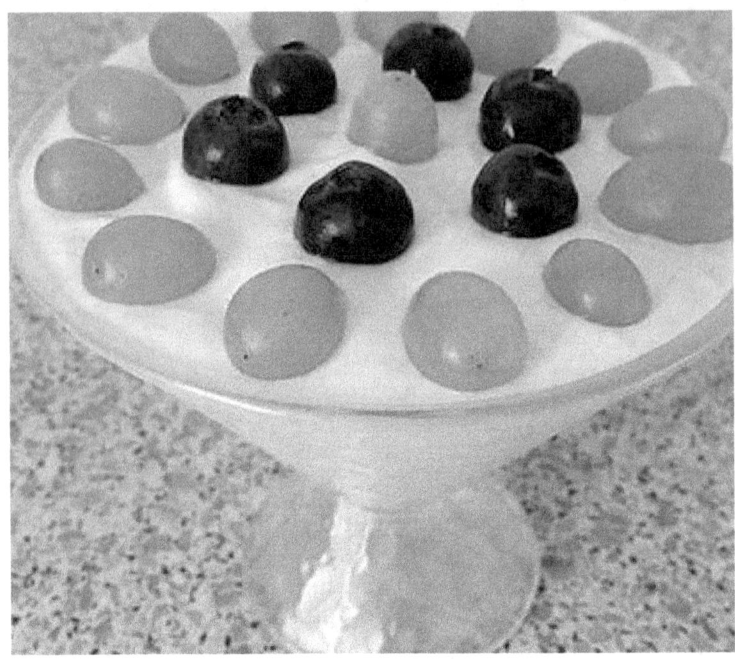

Ingredients for 4 portions

500 ml milk

500 g   low-fat quark

8 ml   Sweetener, liquid, alternatively Stevia

1 pck.   Custard powder

1 splash   Butter and vanilla flavor, optional

Preparation

Total time approx. 15 minutes

Stir custard powder with a little cold milk until smooth. Bring remaining milk to the boil, stir in the stirred powder and bring to a boil while stirring. Remove the vanilla pudding from the heat and stir in the curd cheese until a smooth mass is obtained. Let cool down. Sweetener and who likes, stir in a dash of butter vanilla flavor. DO NOT put the sweetener in the hot pudding, it will lose its taste if it gets too hot.

So you get a light, simple and super delicious cheesecake cream that you can treat yourself even with a diet. I like to eat hot, but it also tastes cold. Including cooking, I'll be ready in 10 - 15 minutes.

CRUMB TUBERS COTTAGE CHEESE

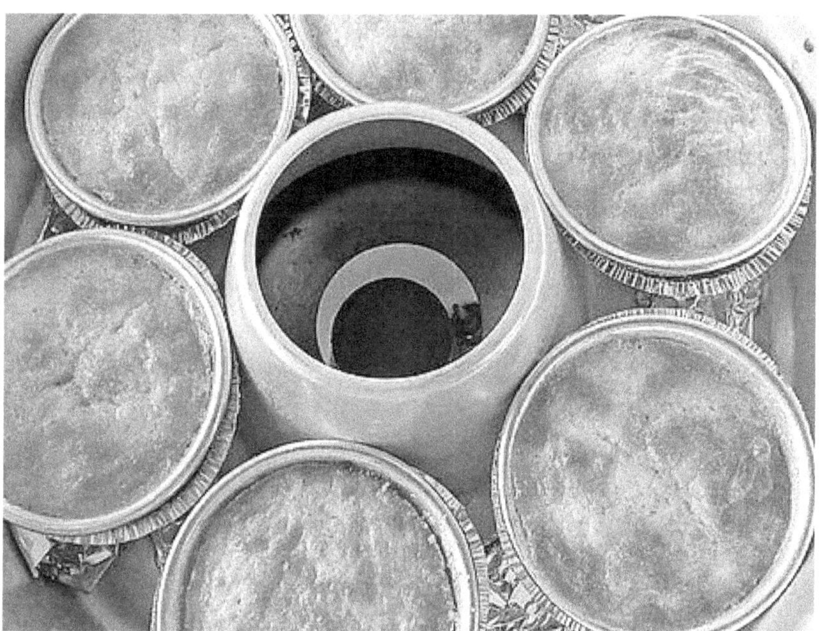

Ingredients for 1 portion

200 g   cottage cheese

10 g   butter

15 g   Flour, (almond flour)

2   Egg

6 splashes   Stevia

2 tsp.   Vanilla, ground

1 tsp.   baking powder

Preparation

Total time approx. 55 minutes

Grease 6 small molds (the size as for muffins) with butter and sprinkle with almond flour.

Mix the eggs, butter, vanilla and stevia thoroughly with a whisk, stir in the cottage cheese, mix the almond flour with the baking powder, add and stir thoroughly. If you like it sweeter, you should work carefully with more stevia.

Baked the whole thing in the molds in an Omnia oven on the gas stove. Baking time 45 minutes. In a normal oven, bake at about 180 degrees with top and bottom heat, for about 35 minutes

QUARK CASSEROLE

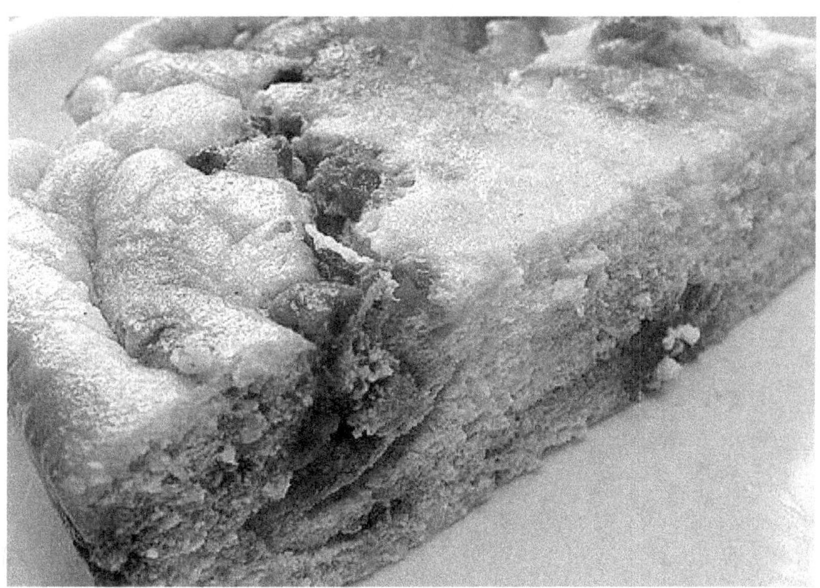

Ingredients for 1 portions

250 g   Quark

1   Egg

3   protein

1 tbsp. semolina

1 tbsp. protein powder

        Fruit of your choice (e.g. berries or apples)

        Sweetener

Preparation

Total time approx. 40 minutes

Beat the egg whites until stiff and mix with the egg, quark, egg white powder and semolina. Sweet with sweetener and bake in a small casserole dish for approx. 30 minutes at 160 degrees.

Depending on your mood you can cover the casserole with berries or apples beforehand.

FROZEN BOUNTY COCONUT CAKE

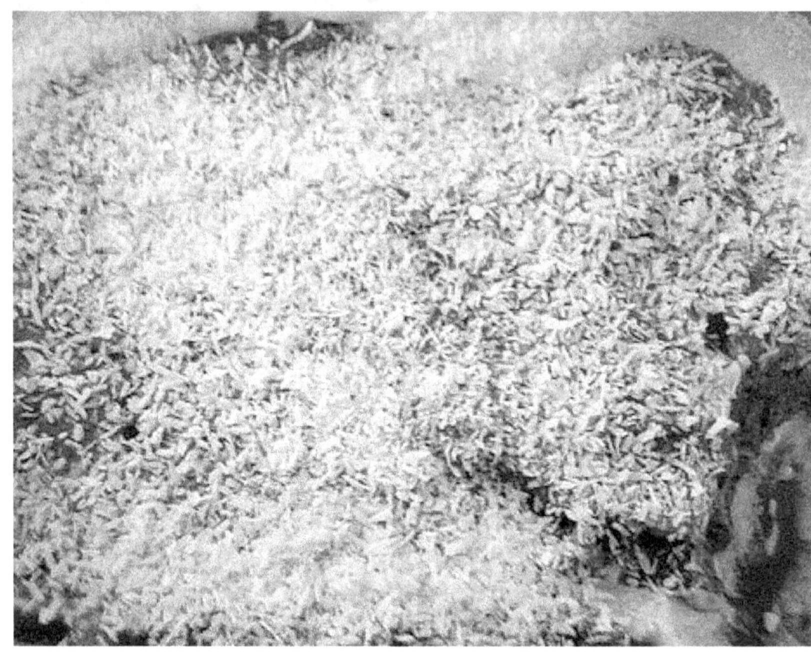

Ingredients for 2 portions

500 ml Yoghurt (coconut yoghurt)

5 Large protein

60 g   Protein powder with vanilla or coconut flavor

20 g	desiccated coconut
15 g	cocoa powder
30 g	Cream cheese
	Sweetener

Preparation

Total time approx. 3 hours 45 minutes

Process the yoghurt with the protein, the protein powder and half of the grated coconut to a homogeneous mass. Add sweetener as needed.

Put half of the mass in a jar.

Mix the remaining half with the cocoa powder and the spread. This now on the first half and sprinkle with the remaining grated coconut.

Put in the freezer for 3 - 4 hours and then serve.

HEAVENLY DESSERT WITH FRUITS

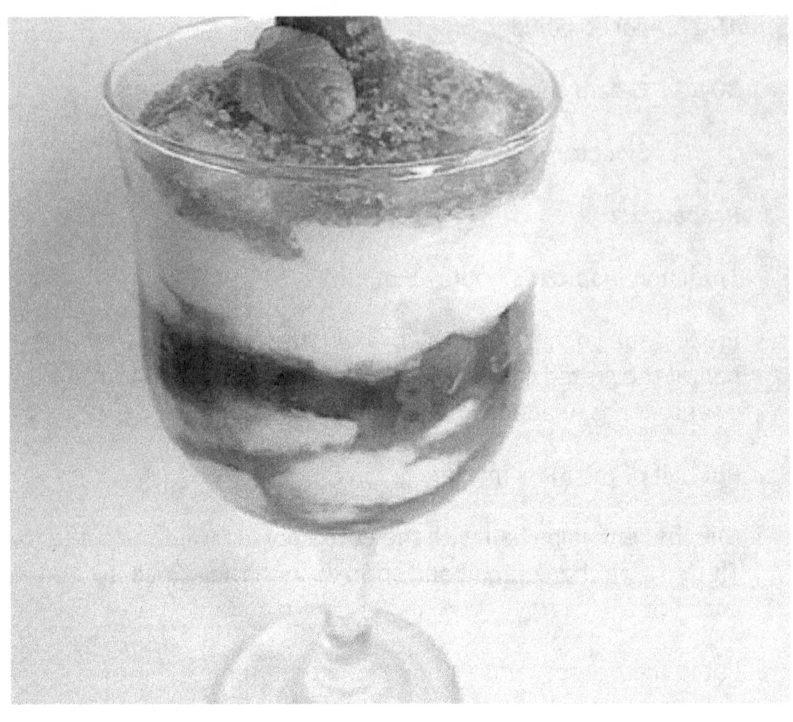

Ingredients for 6 portions

500 g   Raspberries

500 g   Quark (lean quark)

2 cups   whipped cream

2 pck.   Vanilla

         Cane sugar, coarse

Preparation

Total time approx. 15 minutes

Put the raspberries in a bowl or casserole dish (rectangular or round) and distribute.

Now mix curd quark and vanilla sugar with each other. Whip the whipped cream and stir gently under the quark mixture. Distribute the quark cream mixture on the fruit. Now the cane sugar is sprinkled on top - about 3 mm thick.

Put the dessert in the refrigerator for 24 hours until consumption.

STRAWBERRY ICE CREAM

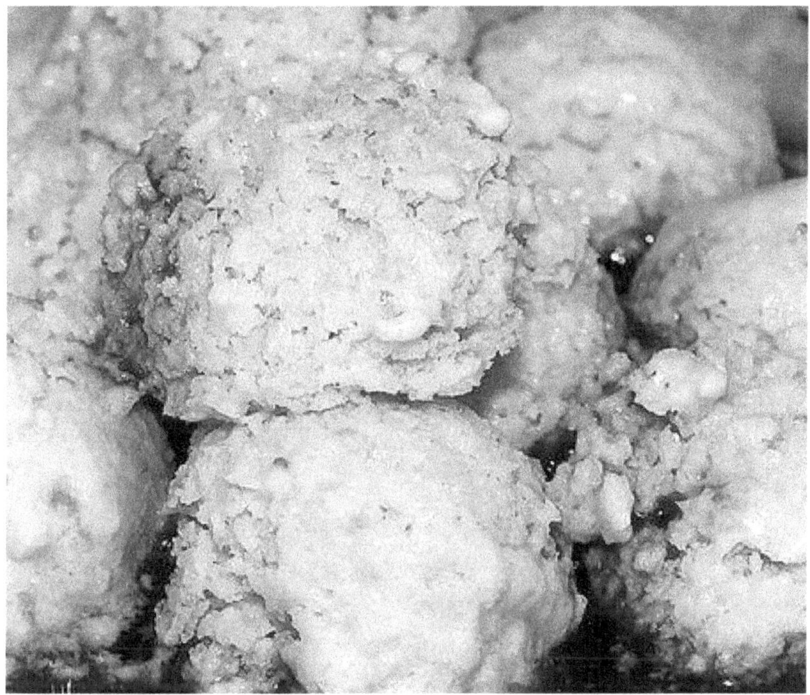

Ingredients for 2 portions

200 g   Strawberries, fresh

200 g   fat yogurt

2 Tea spoons   sugar

1 bag   vanilla sugar

Preparation

Total time approx. 10 minutes

Wash the strawberries and add them to the blender. Add the foam, add the sugar, vanilla sugar and yoghurt and mix until well blended. Then place the mixture in a freezer container and let it solidify in the freezer.

Before serving, thaw the strawberry ice cream briefly and whip up again in the blender. This gives it a soft consistency.

If you want to sweeten this ice cream, you may also add more sugar. The taste is more like a 'water ice' than a 'milk ice'.

CHEESECAKE CREAM

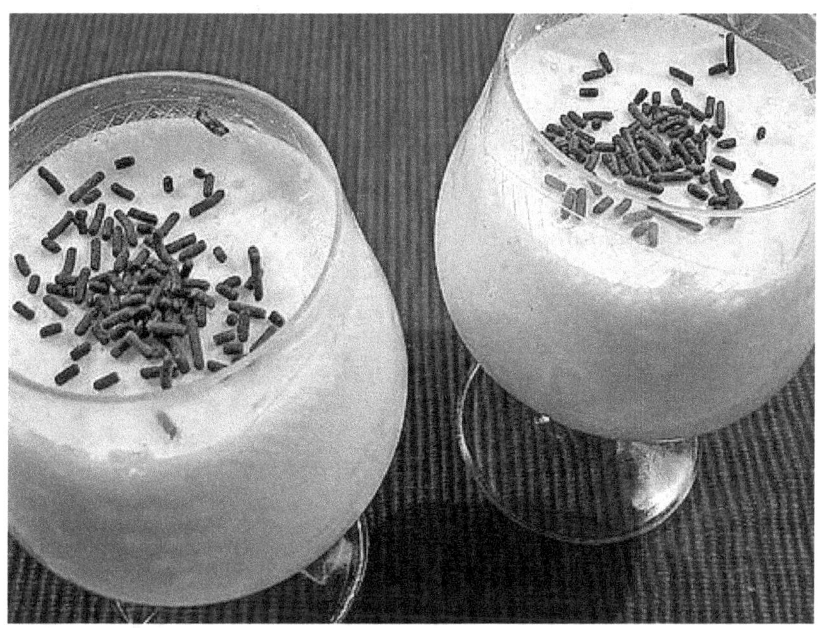

Ingredients for 5 portions

1 bag   Jelly Lemon flavor

500 ml water

500 g   Lean quark (0.2% fat)

2 pck.   Vanilla sugar

1   Vanilla pod, the marrow thereof or 1 pck vanilla sugar

           Stevia

Preparation

Total time approx. 1 hour 45 minutes

Put the stevia powder (dose according to the package instructions) with the vanilla sugar or the marinade of a vanilla pod and the jelly powder together in a large bowl (this should be able to hold the total volume of all ingredients).

Boil 250 ml of water and pour over the powder mixture. Mix well with a whisk until everything has dissolved. Add the remaining 250 ml (cold) water.

Now fold in the quark. Put the whole thing in the freezer for about 45 minutes - 1 hour.

Then remove from the freezer and beat with a whisk until foamy. Put the cream again in the freezer (here you can spread the now foamy mass again on small glass) until the desired consistency is reached.

YOGURT ICE CREAM WITH RHUBARB STRAWBERRY SWIRLS

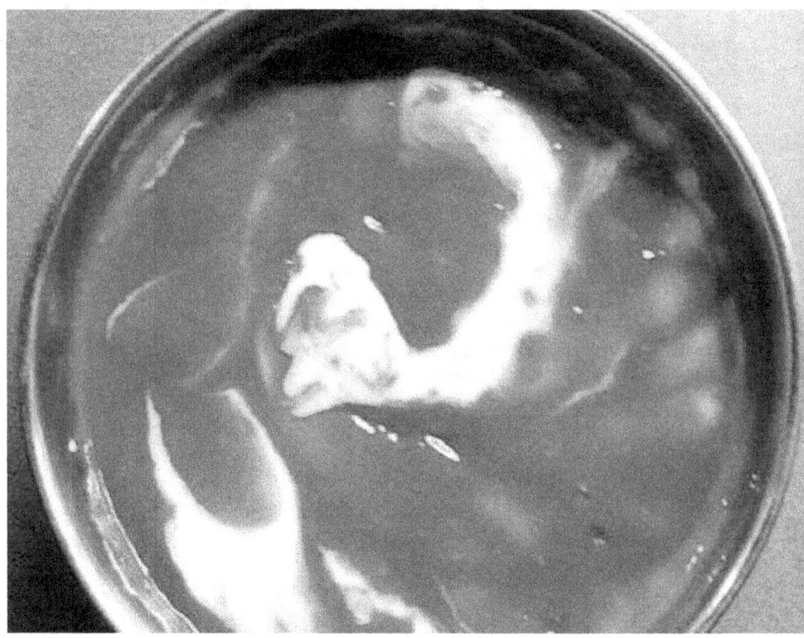

Ingredients for 1 portion

500 g   cream

500 g	Yogurt, 3.5%
120 g	Sweetener, (erythritol)
1 tsp.	vanilla
500 g	strawberries
200 g	rhubarb
	Sweetener, (erythritol)

Preparation

Total time approx. 45 minutes

Heat 100 g of the cream with the erythritol until it has dissolved. Let cool down. Whip in the remaining cream, stir in the yoghurt and vanilla seeds and stir in the cooled cream syrup. Put the mass in the freezer.

Clean and cut the strawberries and rhubarb. Add some erythritol (rather start with a little) and let it boil until it has the consistency of a jam. Season again with sweetener. Let cool down.

The yoghurt ice cream should be stirred well approx. Once an hour so that ice crystals do not form. As soon as the ice has the consistency of soft ice cream (about 3-4 hours), spread the strawberry rhubarb mass evenly and marinate with a spoon. Freeze for at least another hour.

PROTEIN PANCAKE WITHOUT EGG

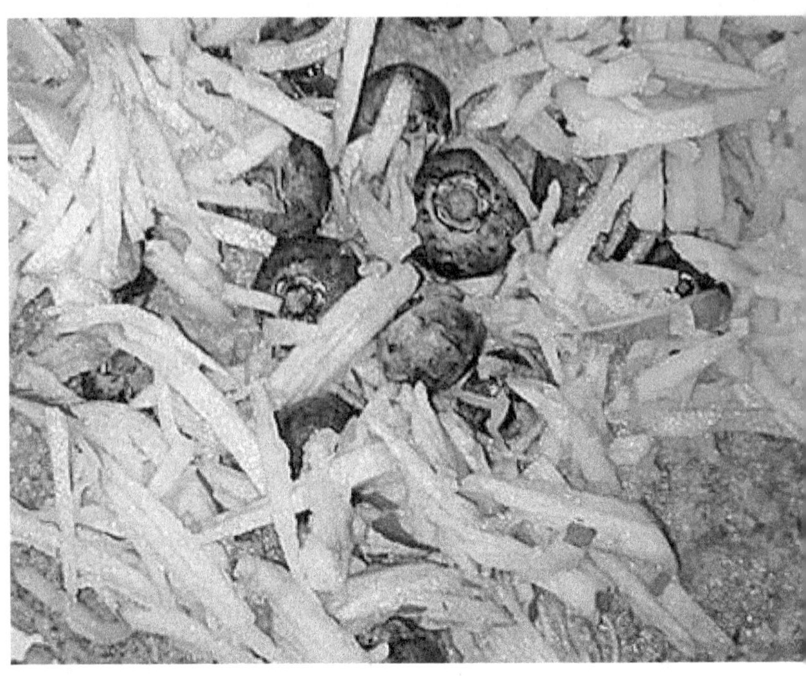

Ingredients for 1 portion

25 g   Powder (protein)

60 ml   Milk, 0.3% fat

1 tbsp. Flax seed, crushed

3 tbsp. water

1 tsp.   psyllium

       Stevia

Possibly.   Cinnamon

     Oil, for frying

Preparation

Total time approx. 30 minutes

Mix the water with the flaxseed meal and let it swell for a few minutes. The mixture is the replacement for an egg.

Then mix all the ingredients together and leave in the fridge for about 15 minutes. Put the dough into the hot pan with a tablespoon, allow to fry for a short time, turn over.

YOGURT PARFAIT WITH CARROT CAKE

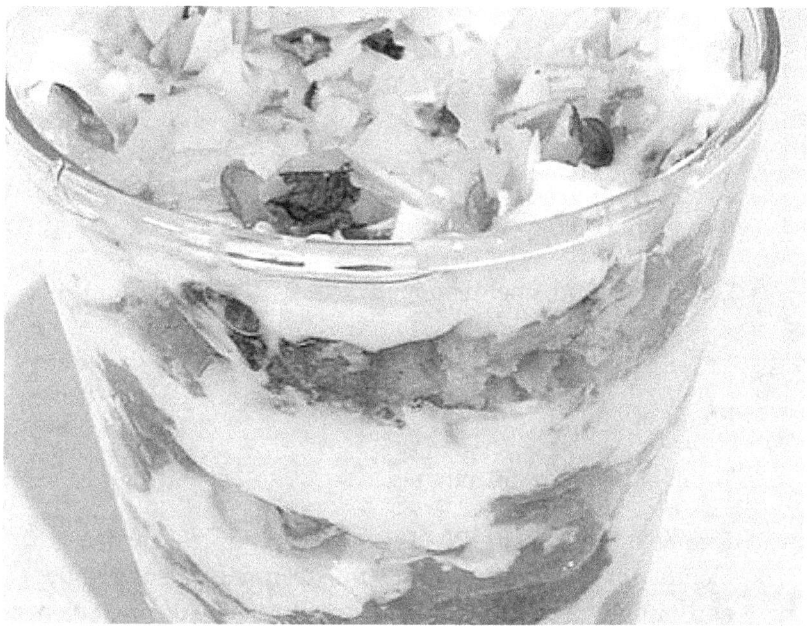

Ingredients for 2 portions

1   Egg

1 tbsp. Stevia

6 tbsp. Almond flour, alternatively ground almonds

55 g   Carrot, peeled and grated

1 teaspoon   baking powder

½ tsp.   cinnamon

½ tsp.   ginger powder

2 pinch salt

½ tsp.   vanilla extract

2 tbsp. Quark

½ tbsp. water

½ tbsp. coconut oil

300 g   Yogurt

½ tbsp. honey

20 g   Almond, finely chopped

20 g   Walnuts, finely chopped

Preparation

Total time approx. 50 minutes

First heat the oven to 170 ° C. Beat eggs and stevia with a
blender for 5-6 minutes or until the mixture thickens slightly
and assumes a light yellow, even color. Mix the dry ingredients
in a bowl and add the egg mixture. Mix cottage cheese and
water and add both to the dough.

Grease a small ovenproof mold with oil. Spread the dough and bake for 20 - 25 minutes. Let the cake cool and then break it into small pieces.

Now take turns adding a layer of cake crumbs, yogurt, honey, almonds and walnuts to a glass.

SUGAR-FREE CARAMEL SAUCE

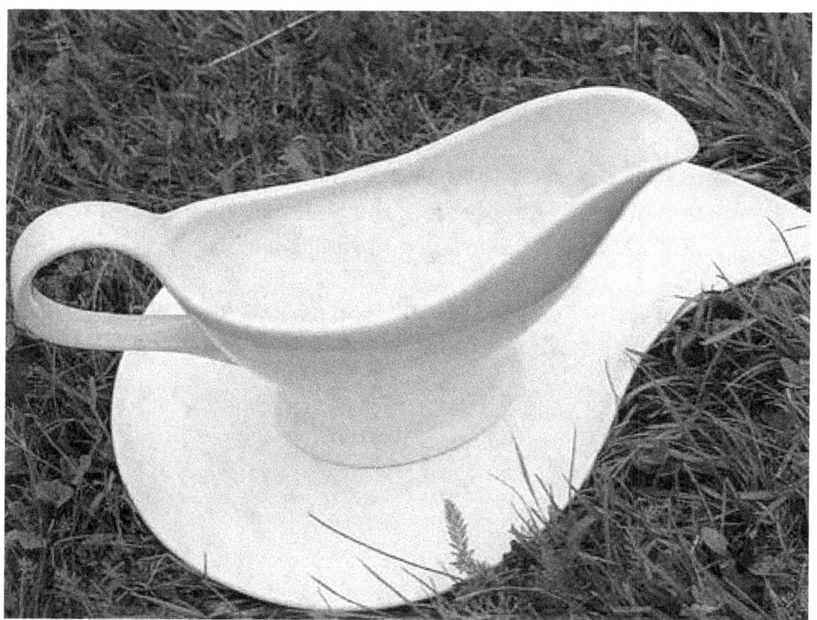

Ingredients for 1 portion

80 ml   water

300 g   Xylitol (sugar substitute), possibly powder sugar

75 g   butter

150 ml   cream

          Vanilla

Salt

Preparation

Total time approx. 30 minutes

Mix powdered sugar with water in a small saucepan.
Alternatively, use sugar in a blender to make powdered sugar.
So he dissolves better and later nothing crystallizes. Heat the
mixture slowly over medium heat. Always stir until the sugar
has dissolved. Bring to a boil and simmer over medium heat for
15 - 20 minutes until the liquid assumes an amber browning.
This can go faster or take longer depending on the power of
your stove. Stir occasionally.

Once the color is reached, add the butter and stir until it has
melted. Remove the pot from the heat and add the cream
carefully and slowly. Finally, add vanilla and salt.

Put the sauce in a glass jar and let it cool down, it will thicken
something else. The caramel sauce stays in the fridge for at
least 2 weeks.

PUDDING BEATEN

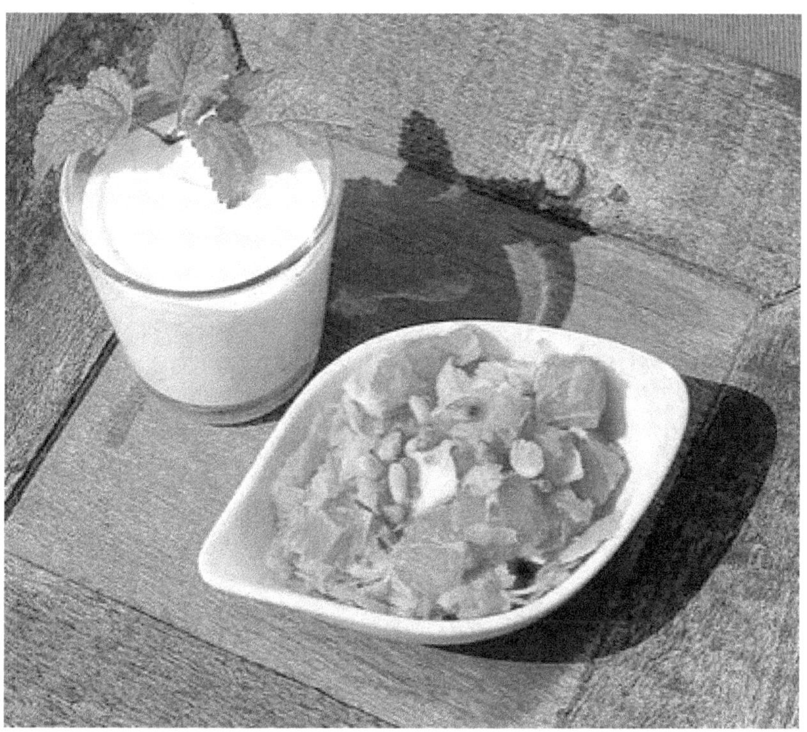

Ingredients for 1 portion

80 ml   Milk, 0.1% fat

2 g   Locust bean gum

            Sweetener

60 g   low-fat quark

125 g   Yogurt, to taste, low in calories

            Fruits, e.g. B from the TC

Preparation

Total time approx. 10 minutes

Skimmed milk, well chilled, beat stiff with carob seed flour for 3 to 4 minutes. Sweet to taste with sweetener and set aside. The mass should taste pure.

Make a cream from skimmed quark, yoghurt and sweetener. Gently lift the first mass under the second. Add to taste, for example, hot berries.

Consume quickly.

FRUITY SUMMER FITNESS MUFFINS WITH MANGO

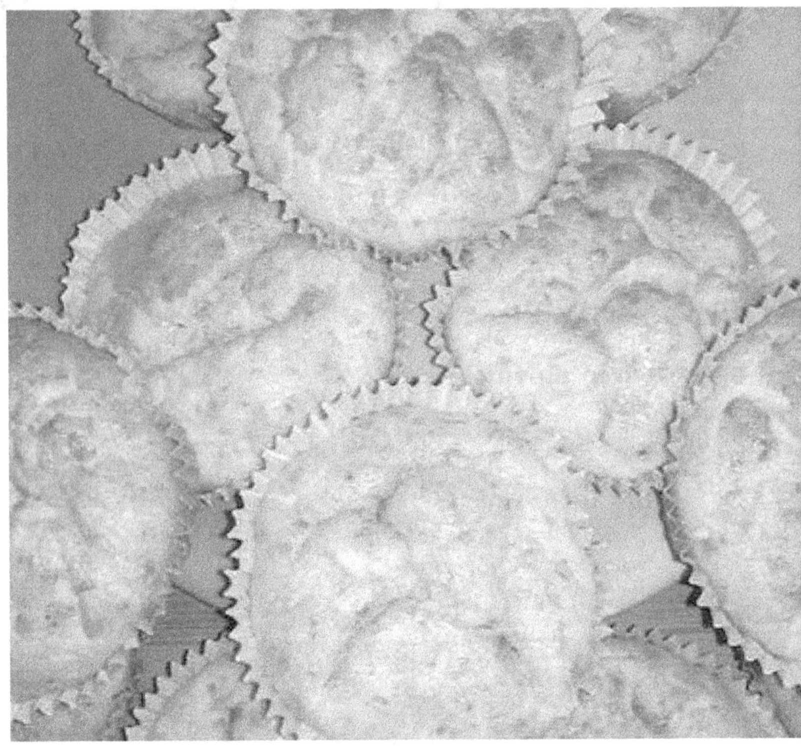

Ingredients for 4 portions

250 g   Lean quark

100 g   Mango, fresh or frozen

30 g   coconut flour

30 g   Wheat bran or spelled bran

50 g   Protein powder, z. B. with banana flavor

3 Large Egg

6 drops Flavdrops e.g. strawberry flavor

3 tbsp. Xylitol (sugar substitute) or another sweetener

Preparation

Total time approx. 1 hour 5 minutes

Mix the dry ingredients and baking powder, then stir in the curd cheese and crushed fruits. Then there are the eggs and sweeteners.

Since I wanted to bake a nice sweet low-carb snack, I chose flavdrops with strawberry flavor and also some erythritol. Of course you can vary that, as well as the choice of protein powder, I only had banana flavor in the house.

Fill the dough into muffin cups and bake at approx. 180 - 200 ° C top / bottom heat for 30 minutes, depending on the oven. Do not get too dark. Allow to cool before eating.

BLUEBERRY PANCAKES MADE FROM ALMOND FLOUR

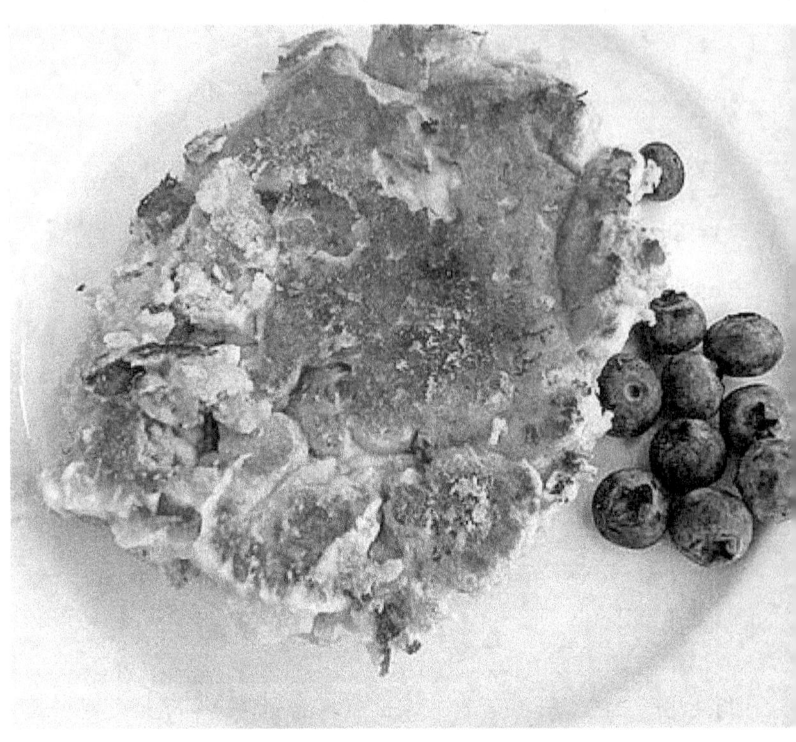

Ingredients for 2 portions

100 g	Almond, ground
60 g	milk
2	Egg
1 teaspoon	baking powder
1 handful	blueberries
	Thick juice (agave), or maple syrup
4 tbsp.	Natural yoghurt
	Sunflower oil

Preparation

Total time approx. 20 minutes

Beat the eggs until frothy. Then add the almond flour, the baking powder and the milk and stir at the lowest level. Leave for a minute.

In the meantime, heat some oil in a frying pan and then fry the pancakes golden-yellow from each side, spoon-by-spoon.

If you want, you can add the blueberries to the dough.

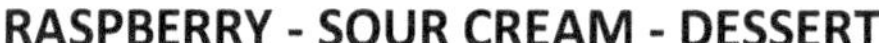

RASPBERRY - SOUR CREAM - DESSERT

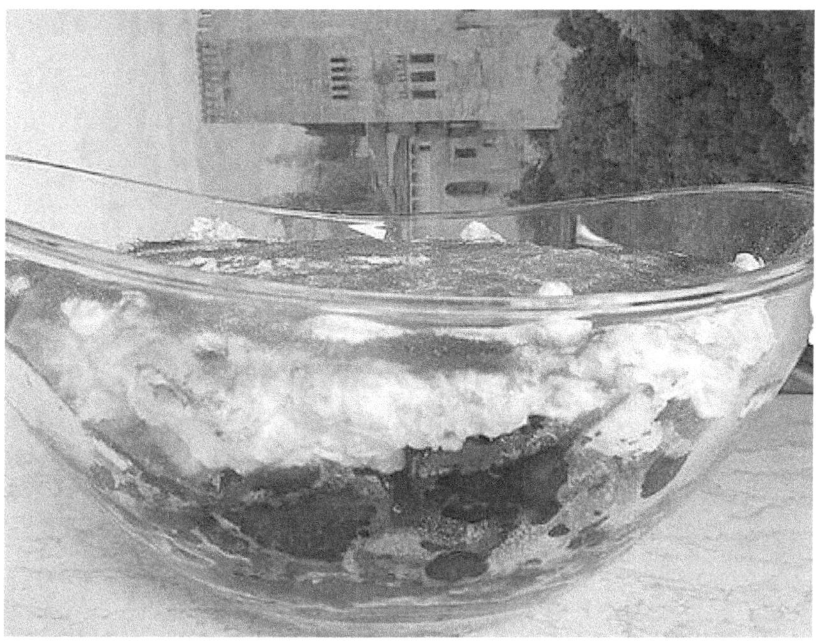

Ingredients for 6 portions

800 g   Raspberries

500 ml cream

2 cups   sour cream

Sugar, brown

Preparation

Total time approx. 8 hours 12 minutes

Frozen raspberries in a flat bowl (baking dish). Beat the cream until stiff, mix with the sour cream and spread on the raspberries. Sprinkle the brown sugar knife back thick over it. Cover in the refrigerator overnight.

Just before serving, sprinkle brown sugar over it again.

Tip: cream and sour cream can be replaced by yoghurt or quark.

ALMOND CREAM - WITH FURTHER PROCESSING TO ALMOND NUT BALLS

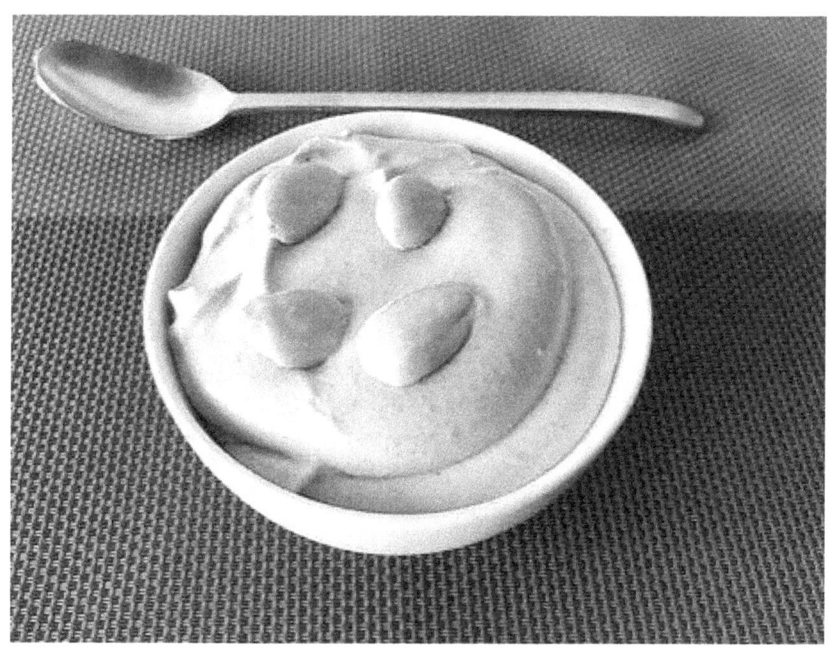

Ingredients for 5 portions

300 g   mascarpone

150 g   Quark

150 g   Almond butter

3 tsp   back cocoa

90 g   Erythritol (sugar replacement)

Furthermore:

450 g   Nuts, chopped, approx., Z. B. hazelnuts, only for the nut balls

Preparation

Total time approx. 3 hours

For the almond cream, mix the mascarpone and cottage cheese in a bowl. Stir in the almond paste, the cocoa and the erythritol. Keep the cream cold for at least 60 minutes. The recipe gives about 5 - 6 servings of cream, each about 100 g or 3 tablespoons.

For the creamy low-carb nut balls, keep the cream cold for 2 hours, the last 30 minutes if necessary in the freezer compartment.

Fill the chopped nuts in a small bowl and roll small balls out of the creamy mass. I recommend about 25 grams of cream per ball. Add this portion to the nuts and roll gently in the nuts, trying to get a spherical shape.

Place the netballs on a plate and cover airtight for 30 minutes.

RASPBERRY ICE CREAM

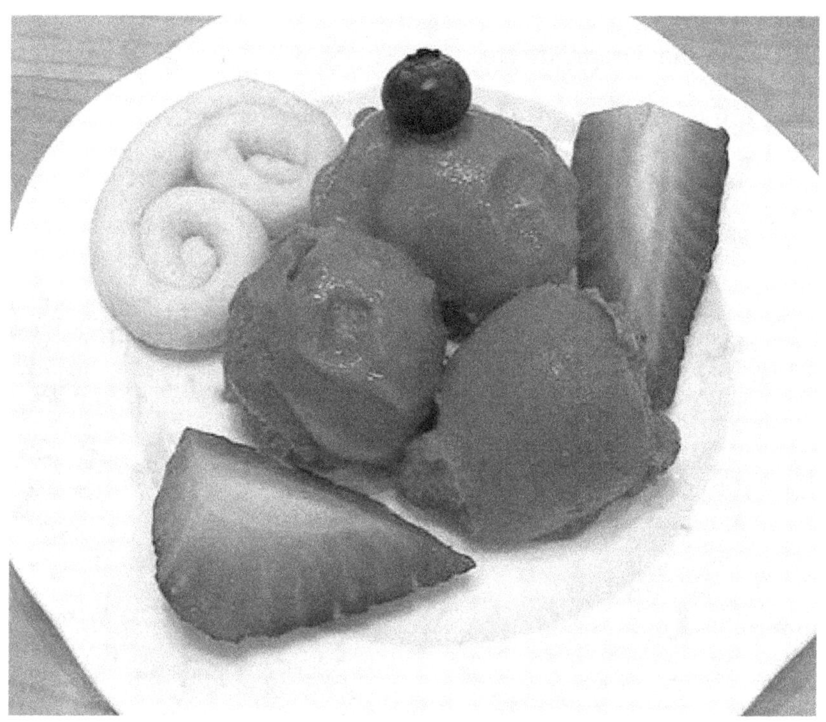

Ingredients for 4 portions

500 g   Raspberries,

400 g   Natural yoghurt 1.5% fat

1 splash   lemon juice

4 small ones   strawberries

Mint leaves

Preparation

Total time approx. 5 minutes

Add the raspberries, lemon juice and yoghurt to the Thermomix and let it run at high speed for 3 - 4 minutes.

Put the finished ice cream in the freezer for another 15 minutes.

To serve, decorate with strawberries and mint leaves.

ALMOND PORRIDGE WITH BERRY SAUCE

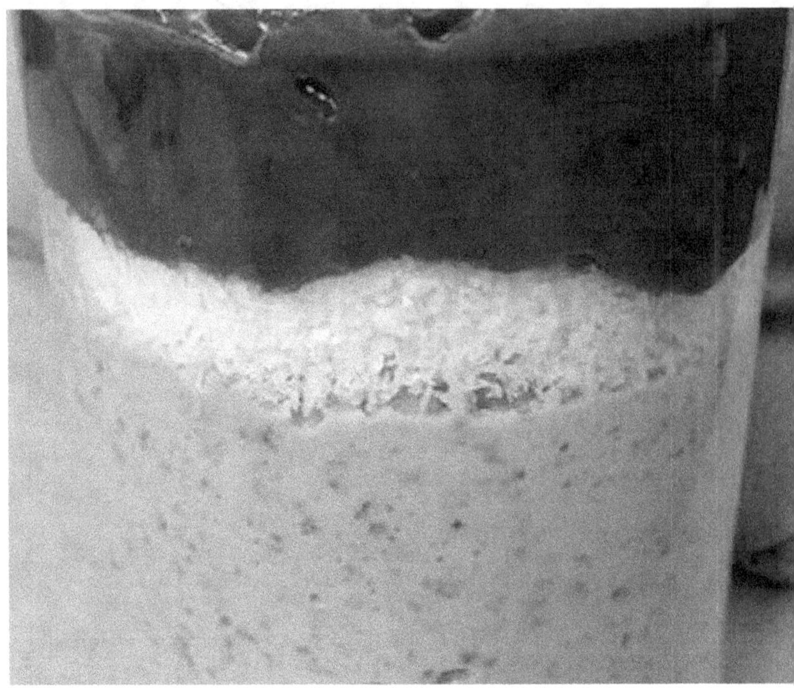

Ingredients for 1 portion

100 ml whipped cream

100 ml water

70 g   Almonds, ground

15 g   desiccated coconut

½ tsp.   Back cocoa

1 teaspoon   Erythritol (sugar replacement)

For the sauce:

50 g   Berries,

1 tbsp. Almond butter

1 teaspoon   Erythritol (sugar replacement)

Preparation

Total time approx. 15 minutes

Slowly bring the cream to a boil with the water.

In another pot also bring the berries to a boil with a little water.

Then stir in the almonds and grated coconut in the cooking cream. Continue stirring until a porridge results. Turn off the heat and add cocoa and erythritol to the porridge.

Add almond purée and erythritol to the simmering berry sauce to make it creamy. Mix the sauce well.

Enjoy the sauce on the porridge and sprinkle coconut flakes or almonds shards as desired.

APPLE VANILLA CHOCOLATE LAYER DESSERT

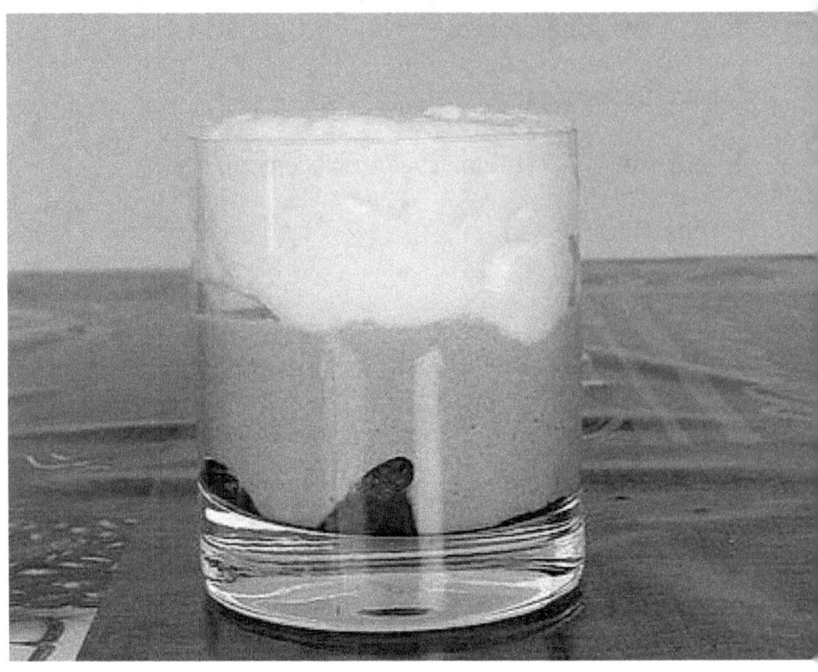

Ingredients for 2 portions

1   Apple

3   protein

250 g   Natural yoghurt, preferably 0.1% fat

1 teaspoon   cocoa powder

3 tsp   Custard powder

Preparation

Total time approx. 10 minutes

Dice the apple and place in two large glasses or on a deep plate.

Stir the cocoa powder into the yoghurt and distribute evenly on the apple.

Beat the egg whites with the mixer until stiff and then stir in the pudding powder. Spread the foam on the yoghurt.

CREAMY COCONUT QUARK

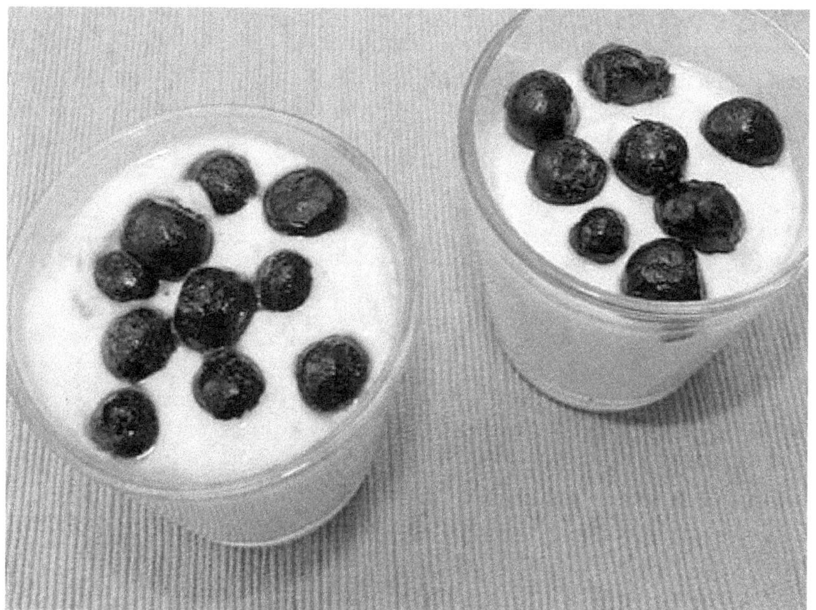

Ingredients for 1 portion

150 g   Quark

80 ml   coconut milk

1 shot   cream

         Vanilla flavor

Sweetener or sugar

Berry

1 teaspoon   Back cocoa

Preparation

Total time approx. 5 minutes

Mix the quark, coconut milk and cream together. Sweet and taste with vanilla flavor.

To refine, add berries or 1 tsp of cocoa at will.

CHOCOLATE CHIA PUDDING

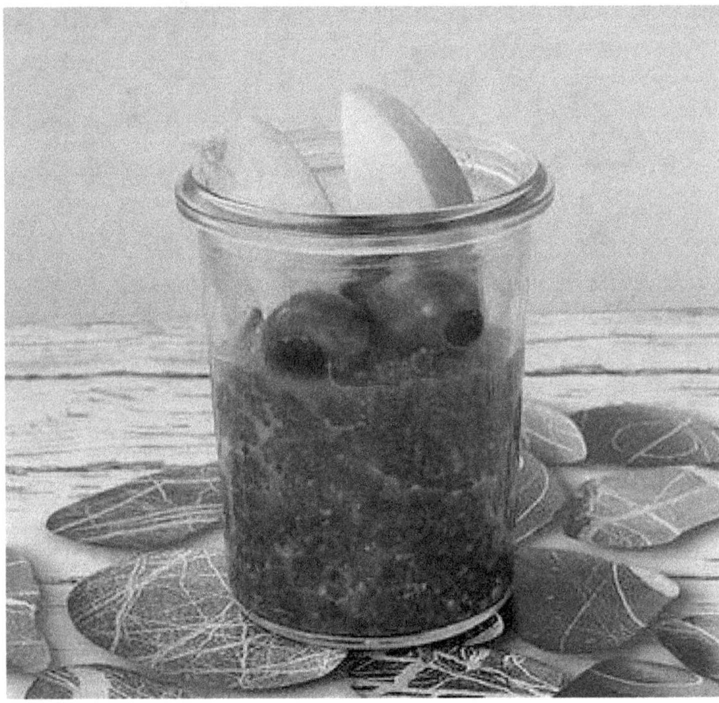

Ingredients for 1 portion

200 ml Almond drink, unsweetened

25 g   Chia seeds

1 teaspoon   cocoa powder

         Sweetener

Preparation

Total time approx. 12 hours 2 minutes

Mix all ingredients together in a sufficiently large (wake-up) glass and stir well. Approximately Let it rest for 10 minutes and then let it soak overnight in the fridge. If desired, the Chia pudding can still be garnished with fresh fruit.

Alternatively, you can modify the pudding to his liking and stir in, for example, 1 teaspoon of cinnamon and a chopped apple or something similar.

QUARK AND RASPBERRY ICE

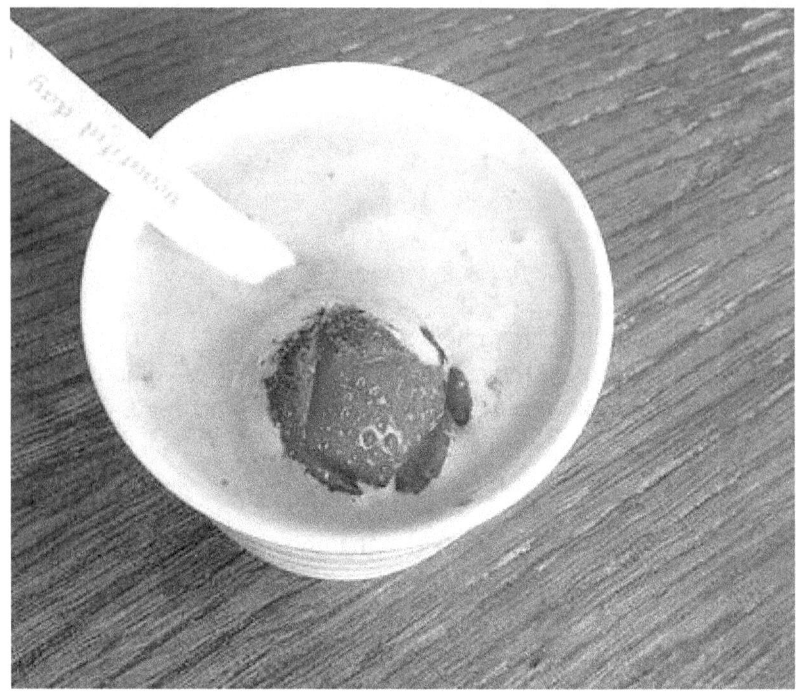

Ingredients for 4 portions

500 g   Raspberries,

400 g   low-fat quark

Possibly.   Honey, 2 - 3 tbsp.

Possibly.   Water

Preparation

Total time approx. 2 hours 10 minutes

Put the frozen raspberries with the cottage cheese in a blender.
Puree the raspberry and quark mixture to a nice smooth mass.
Without honey, the ice cream is actually quite acidic, so if you

like it sweeter, just add 2 - 3 tablespoons of honey in the blender.

If the mass is too thick, add some water or milk. It may be that the mixer does not mix the amount, then just add some liquid, then it should work.

When everything is creamy, divide the ice cream into small bowls and serve. If the ice is still too liquid, simply place it in the freezer for 1 - 2 hours.

If you cannot or do not want to eat everything right away, just freeze it and put it in the microwave for about 1 to 2 minutes before consuming it for the next time. Better too short and in small steps than too long.

PROTEIN OAT CHOCOLATE WAFERS

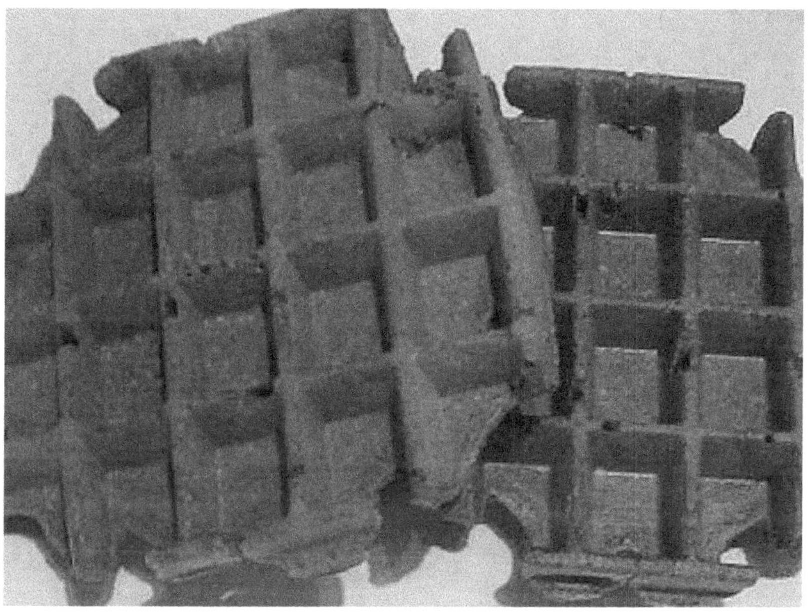

Ingredients for 1 portion

140 g   oatmeal

20 g   Powder (protein)

2   protein

200 g   low-fat quark

4 tbsp. Stevia

2 Tea spoons   cocoa powder

½ Pck.   baking powder

12 drops   Aroma (chocolate sweetener)

1 teaspoon   cinnamon

           Water

Preparation

Total time approx. 25 minutes

Oatmeal in an electric coffee grinder or food processor to process flour. Put all ingredients in a bowl and stir with a little water until a uniform mass is obtained, diluting with water until the dough dries slightly from the spoon.

Bake 1.5 heaped tablespoons per waffle in a waffle iron.

HAZELNUT CREAM

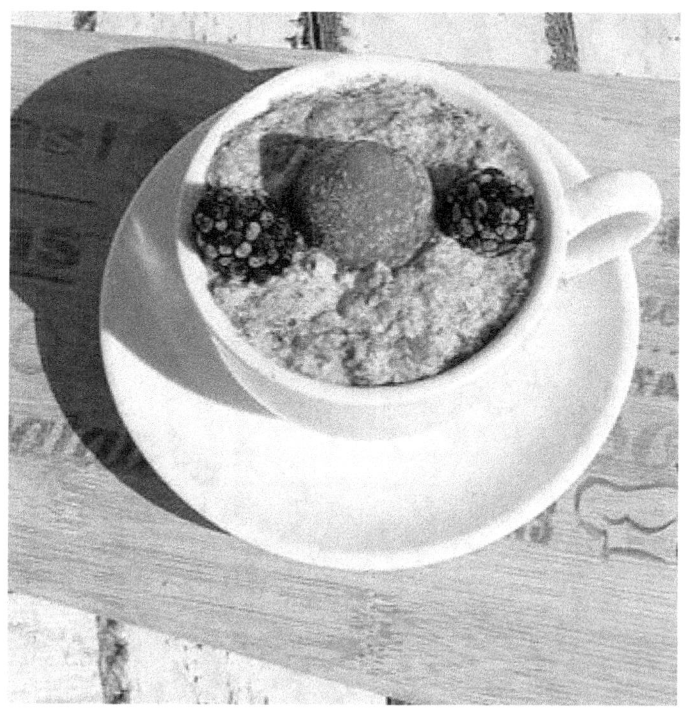

Ingredients for 4 portions

300 ml Soy milk (soy drink), hazelnut milk or almond milk

100 ml cream

200 g   Ground hazelnuts

2 tbsp. Erythritol (sugar replacement)

Preparation

Total time approx. 15 minutes

Bring milk, cream and sugar to a boil in a small saucepan. Add the ground hazelnuts, stir and cook until the cream becomes thicker. Put the cream in a bowl and allow to cool slightly.

Serve warm and Garnish with strawberries.

CHIA FRUIT BREAKFAST

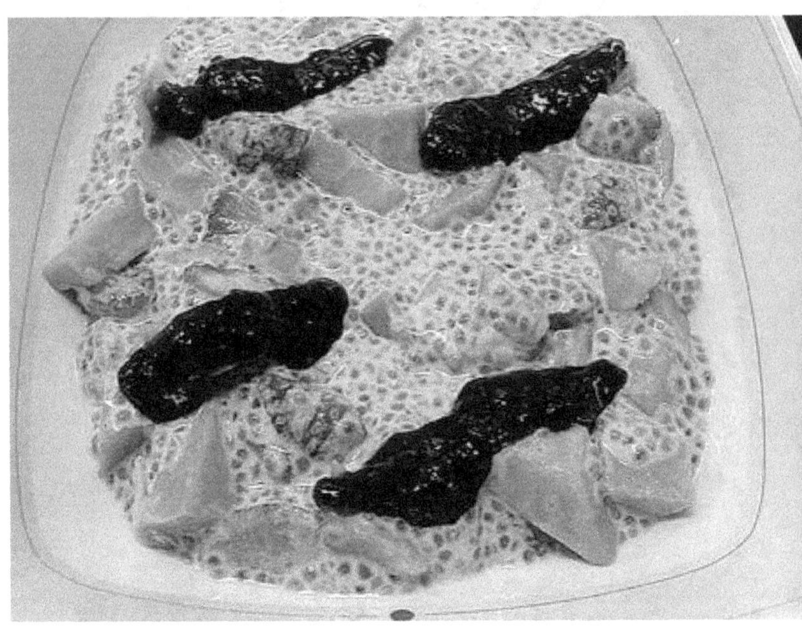

Ingredients for 1 portion

3 tbsp. Chia seeds, processed to gel, see my recipe Chia gel

3 tbsp. coconut milk

1 teaspoon   Xylitol (sugar replacement)

1 pinch cinnamon

        Vanilla, ground

Some   Strawberries or blueberries

        Papaya

        Fruit purée, cold-stirred, optional

Preparation

Total time approx. 5 minutes

The chia gel with the coconut milk and the sugar stir until the sugar dissolves. Add cinnamon and vanilla.

Wash the berries and cut them if necessary. Peel the papaya and cut into pieces, quantity as needed.

RASPBERRY AND MASCARPONE DESSERT

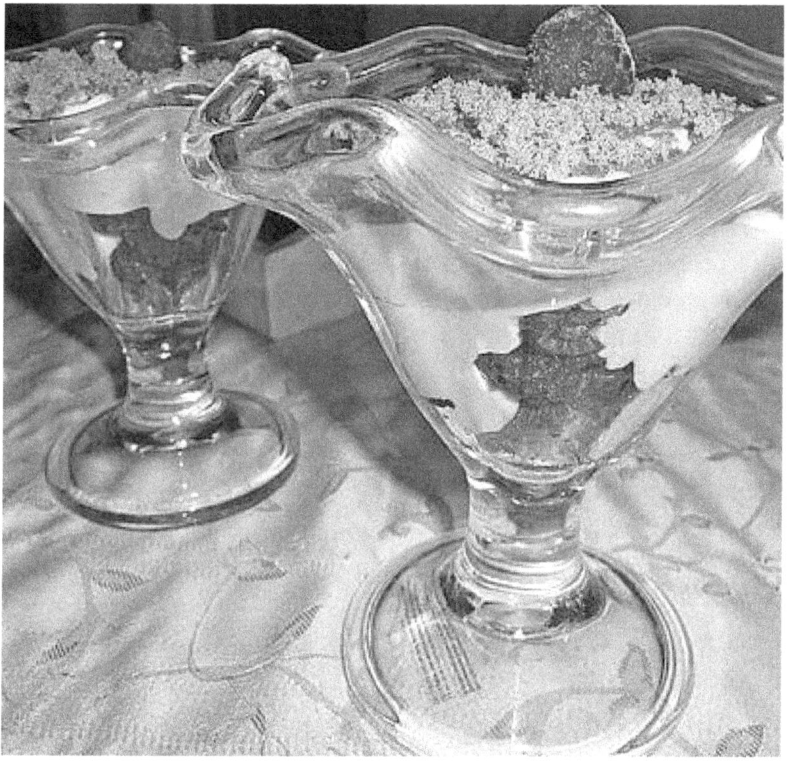

Ingredients for 6 portions

600 g   Raspberries, fresh or frozen

500 g   mascarpone

100 ml coconut milk

50 g   desiccated coconut

1   Vanilla pod (es), scratched marrow thereof

            Vanilla sugar

            Sugar, brown

Preparation

Total time approx. 10 minutes

If necessary, the raspberries are thawed in the sieve and placed in a casserole dish or the like at the bottom spread. Glass is especially pretty here because you can see the layers.

The mascarpone is stirred smoothly with the coconut milk, the coconut flakes, the vanilla pulp and vanilla sugar and then poured over the raspberries. Finally, brown sugar is sprinkled over the cream, creating a sweet layer.

RASPBERRY CREAM WITH WHITE CHOCOLATE

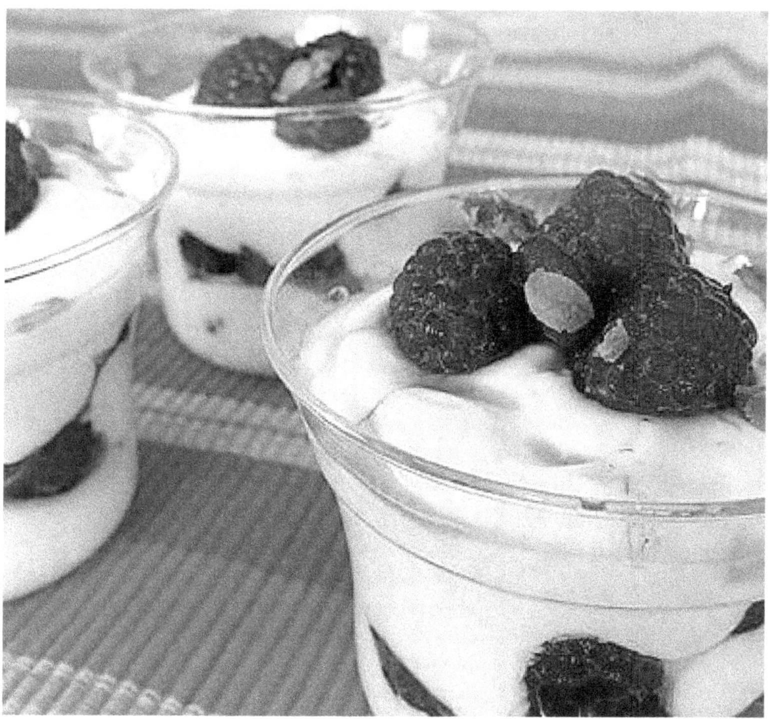

Ingredients for 6 portions

2 cups   sour cream

2 cups   Crème fraiche Cheese

200 g   Chocolate, white

1 bag   Raspberries,

Preparation

Total time approx. 10 minutes

Melt chocolate in a water bath. Mix with sour cream and crème fraiche, chill. Give raspberries over it.

The chocolate toppings can be prepared well the day before.

Freeze the raspberries frozen to the mass and serve when thawed.